616·072
TOLLISON, C David

Managing chronic pain – A patient's
guide 82

83110327

pen marks noted 21/7/92
PMG.

MANAGING CHRONIC PAIN:

A PATIENT'S GUIDE

MANAGING
CHRONIC PAIN:
A PATIENT'S GUIDE

C. David Tollison, Ph.D.

 Sterling Publishing Co., Inc.   New York

To my parents, Wade A. Tollison and Louise J. Tollison,
and my wife, Linda, and children, Courtney and David

I would like to extend a special thank you to Rose-Marie
Strassberg, whose judicious and concerned editing
brought this book to its final publishable state.

All drawings by Bonnie Adamson.

Library of Congress Cataloging in Publication Data

Tollison, C. David, 1949–
    Managing chronic pain.

    Includes index.
    1. Pain—Treatment.   2. Chronically ill—Rehabilita-
tion.   I. Title.   [DNLM: 1. Pain—Therapy—Popular works
WL 704 T651m]
RB127.T63   616′.0472   81-85035
ISBN 0-8069-5570-8   AACR2
ISBN 0-8069-5571-6 (lib. bdg.)

Contents

God whispers to us in our pleasures, speaks in our conscience, but shouts in our pains . . .

C.S. Lewis
"The Problem of Pain"

CHAPTER ONE

What Is Pain?

Perhaps Charlie Brown, in the "Peanuts" comic strip, defined pain best when he declared, "Pain is when it hurts." Few doctors can agree on a definition much beyond that, because pain can vary so dramatically from one person to another or from one part of the body to another. We all have experienced pain at some point in our lives, and we all know what it feels like to hurt. Yet, our language really does not permit us to define pain accurately. Even scientifically, with all we know about pain mechanisms, neuropsychology and neurophysiology, the phenomenon of pain eludes a clear definition.

We do know that pain has always been part of the human condition and is a major concern influencing every aspect of life. In fact, pain is the single most common symptom which compels us to seek medical counsel. The advent of science brought a new approach to pain, that of seeking to understand its origins and outcomes in a rigorous way and of identifying systematic methods for alleviating the misery associated with it. People have used potions, magic and pain-relieving remedies for centuries, but the search for treatment based on controlled scientific investigation is a recent development. The scientific search for answers to the problems of pain has provided doctors and other health professionals with a wealth of information to use in helping us learn to manage pain in positive ways. Yet, much still remains to be learned.

Acute vs. Chronic Pain

In general terms, there are two types of pain: acute and chronic. All of us have experienced acute pain at some time in our lives, whether the result of slamming an automobile door on a finger, falling off a skateboard, or some other daily activity that suddenly "goes wrong." Acute pain serves as a warning that something somewhere in our body is amiss and requires immediate attention. A headache may last all day, and a sprained ankle may hurt for a week. Nevertheless, acute pain does have a time limit. The discomfort may be severe, but we know that the pain will be alleviated in time.

Acute pain also serves a protective function. A finger accidentally placed on a hot oven will produce an instantaneous "jerk-reflex" as the hand is quickly removed. The finger may blister and cause extreme pain, but there is really little to worry about. Acute pain, by definition, gets better.

Table 1–1

COMPARISON OF ACUTE AND CHRONIC PAIN

Acute Pain	Chronic Pain
Useful	Little significance
Brief duration	More than six months' duration
Well-defined and usually successful treatment	Multifactorial treatment and with limited success
Limited drug therapy with few complications	Prolonged drug therapy with many complications
Sympathy is appropriate	Sympathy may be inappropriate
No permanent disability	Permanent management

When pain persists for six months or more, it is considered chronic in nature. Chronic pain does not serve as a warning for the body to take action. In fact, unlike acute pain, chronic pain serves no useful purpose whatsoever. Whereas acute pain can usually be tied to a source, the causes of chronic pain are often uncertain. While acute pain is a symptom of some injury, disease or disorder, chronic pain is more correctly described as a disease itself, rather than a symptom of something else. Whereas acute pain, by definition, gets better, chronic pain may never heal and, in fact, often gets steadily worse. Chronic pain can be continuous, 24 hours a day, seven days a week, 365 days a year. While the intensity of the discomfort may vary—sometimes worse, sometimes not as bad—one factor remains constant: The pain is *always* present.

The Cost of Pain

Pain is an enormous social and personal problem, one that all of us must encounter occasionally and one that chronic-pain victims must cope with every day of their lives. Low-back pain, for example, will afflict eight of every ten Americans at some time during their lives, regardless of their sex or age. For many of these sufferers, the pain will persist for months and even years. Chronic pain is today an unrecognized epidemic in this country, ranking behind only cancer and heart disease in the number of persons afflicted with disease.

Estimated expenditures on the treatment of pain in the United States increased from threefold to fivefold between 1976 and 1981. We can calculate doctor and hospital costs, analgesic drug (drugs used to relieve pain) costs, and disability/compensation payments. However, there is no means to accurately calculate the cost to industry in personnel replacement costs and lost productivity.

Most authorities agree that approximately eight to 12 percent of the American population suffers chronic pain. The *Journal of Occupational Health and Safety* (45: 1976) reports that "on any given day, approximately eight million workers are under treatment for chronic pain resulting from an industrial accident or injury. As such, chronic pain represents the most frequent industrial disabler." In fact, chronic low-back pain, frequently the result of an industrial injury, represents the single most costly malady in the 30-to-60-year age group. Some authorities believe that over 700 million workdays a year are lost because of pain. The cost to industry for this lost productivity is enormous and is ultimately passed on to the consumer.*

The average chronic-pain sufferer in the United States has suffered for seven years, undergone three to five major surgeries, and spent from $50,000 to $100,000 in doctors' bills

*M. Feuerstein & E. Skjei, *Mastering Pain* (New York: Bantam Books, 1979), p. 3.

alone.* At least ten billion dollars are spent annually by sufferers of serious pain for prescription analgesic drugs or surgical procedures and loss to the economy because of time spent away from their jobs.** Forty million people in this country suffer from recurrent headaches. Millions of dollars' worth of nonprescription, over-the-counter medicines are sold that provide only temporary relief.

The *total* annual expenditure on treatment of chronic pain in the United States is 60 to 70 *billion* dollars! By comparison, the annual expenditure for treatment of alcoholism, a far more publicized disease, is approximately 30 billion dollars.* Chronic pain represents a serious social, personal and economic epidemic in this country, and the enormous costs in dollars and human suffering continue to rise.

Chronic-Pain Myths

There are a number of myths surrounding the disease of chronic pain. Some misconceptions result from confusing acute pain with chronic pain. Others may be associated with the reluctance of many individuals to accept the fact that such an unpleasant and physical sensation as pain is partially influenced by psychological variables. Still others may be the result of a lack of knowledge of chronic pain, both by doctors and the general public. Here are some common chronic-pain myths:

1. It's all in your head.
2. Psychology has nothing to do with pain.
3. Doctors don't care about pain.
4. Pain is pain—it's all the same.
5. The right drug will cure my pain.
6. Surgery always cures the cause of pain.
7. You don't look sick. How could you have chronic pain?
8. Rest will cure chronic pain.
9. Chronic pain is a disabling disorder.
10. If you ignore it, the pain will go away.
11. Chronic pain can usually be cured.

*Mastering Pain, p. 3.
**Newsweek, April 25, 1977.

12. You deserve to be in pain because you haven't lived a "good" life.
13. My doctor is almost God. He can cure anything.
14. Nobody ever hurt as much as I.
15. All doctors are incompetent.
16. I can't live in pain the rest of my life.
17. My pain affects no one but me.
18. Pain is the result of being physically overactive.
19. Seeing someone in worse shape will make you feel better.
20. You can't do housework or hold a job if you have chronic pain.
21. Chronic pain is always a symptom that something somewhere in your body is "wrong."
22. If a cause for pain can be found, then the pain can be cured.

The Chronic-Pain Patient: A Case History

Frank S. is a chronic-pain patient. He's had neck, low-back and radiating pain down the right leg for four years after falling from a ladder at work and landing on his back. Frank is 51 years old, has a high-school education, is married, and has four grown children.

At the time of Frank's injury, he was taken to the first-aid station where he was attended to by a nurse. Frank initially reported his injury as minor and insisted on returning to work. The nurse approved his return to work under the condition that he report to her several times daily for treatment. Frank tried to work, but the increase in pain when bending created a situation which justified his sitting down to rest. He soon looked forward to visiting the nurse several times daily. The gentle massage made him feel better, and he enjoyed the attention he was receiving.

After several weeks, Frank's pain was no better. The nurse referred him to a surgeon who hospitalized him, ordered bed rest and prescribed muscle relaxants and analgesics. Frank also had X rays taken which did not show anything unusual, yet his pain persisted. After several days, Frank's surgeon started traction and physical therapy. These treatments seemed to relieve the pain temporarily, but soon the discomfort was again severe.

The doctor tried changing the medication regimen, each time increasing the dosage and potency of the drugs. Frank received no relief from pain but did notice a welcomed change in his wife. To his surprise, she was showing concern and even anxiety about his health. He also enjoyed the frequent visits of his children, who drove long distances almost daily to pamper him.

In time, Frank was discharged from the hospital and told to stay home from work, take the drugs prescribed, and to return for an office visit in two weeks. He followed the doctor's orders completely and returned at the appointed time, reporting a recent *increase* in pain. The surgeon again hospitalized Frank, this time for a myelogram and electrodiagnostic studies, which indicated two ruptured discs in the lower back. Surgery was performed, and everyone—including Frank—believed the days of constant pain were almost over.

Unfortunately, relief did not come. Frank continued to have pain following surgery. The surgeon called in a variety of specialists, none of whom could explain why the pain was still present. Frank was frustrated and convinced that his surgeon was a "quack." He went home from the hospital, swallowed analgesics by the handful, stayed in bed, and became increasingly depressed. He also became irritable, and his wife, children and friends gradually decreased their solicitous visitations.

Frank consulted another doctor who believed the cause of pain was a trapped nerve root. Surgery was again performed with high expectations for pain relief. Unfortunately, the result was the same, and Frank continued to suffer. This time he left the hospital with more analgesic drugs and returned home, even more frustrated, depressed and believing that returning to work was completely out of the question.

Frank is now convinced of his disability. Workmen's compensation verifies this belief with regular monthly disability payments. As a result, there is little incentive to return to work.

In the years to follow, Frank looks forward to appointments with his doctors, partly because they are the only diversion in an otherwise boring day, and partly because it is somehow amusing to defy the doctors' medical expertise. The doctors readily admit they do not know what else to try, so they continue giving Frank drugs which are enjoyed because of the resulting emotional lift. Five or ten years from now, the situation will likely remain unchanged. Maybe the doctors and drugs will be different, but the pattern of life will remain the same. Frank has fallen victim to the chronic-pain trap.

CHAPTER TWO

The Biphasic
Nature of Pain

Before the early part of the nineteenth century, the phenomenon of pain was viewed as an essentially emotional event. This concept had for many centuries changed little from that expressed in the early dissertations of Aristotle, who considered pain in the category of an emotion—specifically, the opposite of pleasure. Aristotle believed that pain was more an appropriate topic for philosophical study than a consideration for physicians.

With the advances of science and the explosion of knowledge concerning the structure and function of the human body, neurophysiology and neurology increasingly challenged these philosophical ideas and ultimately succeeded in establishing the importance of considering pain a physiological phenomenon. Much interest has subsequently been generated in clarifying the nature of pain in physiological terms. While no theoretical model has yet been devised that can account for all the experimental and clinical observations concerning it, there is widespread agreement among researchers in the field of pain, especially chronic pain, that the phenomenon we call pain is much more complex than traditional physiological explanations would suggest. In fact, chronic pain is today considered a complex subjective perception composed of at least *two* major components: physiology and psychology.

PHYSIOLOGICAL MECHANISMS OF PAIN

Physiological Structure and Function

The perception of pain involves the entire central nervous system: the brain, spinal cord and miles of nerves in the body. The central nervous system controls the *voluntary* muscles such as those used in walking, picking up a pencil, combing your hair and playing tennis. The phenomenon of pain also involves the sympathetic nervous system, a part of the autonomic nervous system. The autonomic nervous system controls the "automatic," or *involuntary* muscles such as the heart muscle and the muscles that dilate and contract the pupils in your eyes. The sympathetic nerves travel to all the arteries in the body which, in turn, control the amount of blood flow to the muscles.

Nerves serve an important function in the body since they act as pain receptors, picking up pain messages much like a radio antenna picks up radio waves. Pain begins as a stimulus, which is then picked up by nerves. Once a pain stimulus or message is received by a nerve ending, it is carried to the brain and back again to the affected body part by the nerves. Some nerves are single strands of fibre while others are bundled together. Some nerves are coated with a substance called myelin while others are not. Myelin acts as a protective insulation for the electrical charges of nerves.

Nerves are made up of tiny nerve cells which receive and forward pain messages. Each cell has a receiver end called a dendrite and a transmitter end called an axon. Pain messages travel as an electrical impulse from the axons of one cell to the dendrites of the next, and so on down the line. The gap between the axons and dendrites is called a synapse, and it is here that pain messages are deciphered and coded. Depending on the type of coding, a pain message reaching a synapse may be terminated completely, changed and rerouted in some way, or simply forwarded to the neighboring cell.

This "decision at the synapse" is influenced strongly by chemical substances called neurotransmitters that are activated by pain messages. Neurotransmitters also assist in the pain-message transmission since they "bridge the gap" between axons and dendrites. A number of different neurotransmitters have been identified, including serotonin, dopamine, norepinephrine and acetylcholine. This transmission process, however, can be reduced or increased by drugs. In fact, many drugs are purposely designed to alter the transmission of electrical impulses across the synapse.

Many researchers believe that pain messages travel to the brain on one of two "superhighways." The pain message starts with a stimulus and travels up the spinal cord. This highway is called the spinothalamic tract. Once the message gets to the brain, it meets a fork in the road. One highway travels through portions of the brain called the thalamus and hypothalamus to the limbic system. This highway is called the paleospinothalamic tract. This is the tract on which pain that's been described as a steady-ache or dull-ache travels. The other highway is called the neospinothalamic tract. Sharp, stabbing impulses usually travel this highway to the brain.

Biochemistry of Pain

A current topic of interest and debate in scientific circles is the role of biological chemicals in the experience of pain. Unfortunately, there exists much theory, but little fact. In the past few years, most investigative efforts have focussed on the importance of protein substances called neurokinins and the role they play in reducing pain thresholds. Many researchers believe that the experience of pain triggers the release of neurokinins in the body, increasing the discomforting quality of pain. A simple way to think of the role of neurokinins is to imagine a dam and reservoir. Under most conditions, neurokinins are safely stored in the body much like water backed up by a dam. However, under certain conditions, such as heavy and prolonged rain, the dam can break, causing flooding and greatly complicating a bad situation. When pain is experienced, there is not only the problem of discomfort, but the pain may "break the dam" and release a flood of neurokinins, which in turn increase the pain.

One neurokinin theory postulates that the substances are released when tissue cells are damaged or destroyed. The release of neurokinins then concentrates around nerve endings and fibres involved in the transmission of pain signals from a body part to the brain. As the pain message travels up a nerve, neurokinins "amplify" the pain signal.

A similar process has been known to occur in migraine headaches. In the early stage of migraine development, another biochemical, serotonin, is released in the body. Serotonin causes vasoconstriction (arteries in the head decrease their diameter and allow less blood flow). Constriction of the cephalic arteries (located in the head area) and decreased blood flow is thought by many researchers to cause the "flashing lights" and uneasy, light-headed feeling known as prodromals that many migraine victims suffer prior to the onset of severe pain. Once the serotonin is depleted, however, the arteries become more flexible, the body is flooded with a release of neurokinins, and the arteries dilate in throbbing, excruciating pain. The presence of neurokinins is thought to lower the threshold at which the throbbing arterial dilations are felt as painful.

Endorphins

Not only does the body manufacture biochemicals that amplify the intensity of pain (such as neurokinins), but recent research has also identified pain-reducing biochemicals produced in the human body. The name given to these substances is endorphins, and many researchers believe they represent an important component of the body's own mechanism for controlling pain.

Endorphins have a number of similarities to potent narcotic analgesic drugs such as morphine (Chapter Five). For example, endorphins are nearly identical to morphine in molecular structure. In addition, endorphins, like morphine, exert their chemical action by blocking a number of important transmission sites in the central nervous system. This alteration in nerve transmission seems to decrease the intensity and quality of pain. Finally, endorphins are thought to act on the same special cells in the brain and spinal cord that the opiate narcotic drugs attach to in order to produce an analgesic and euphoric effect. Commonly known as opiate receptor cells, these cells seem to have a special affinity for man-made narcotic drugs. This affinity has led researchers to suspect the existence of endorphins even before they were formally identified.

If you seem to have a lower threshold for pain than other people, perhaps your body has a deficiency of endorphins or receptor cells. Research in this area is continuing to document the important role of endorphins in the experience of pain. Endorphins may be prescribed someday to treat chronic pain, depression and other related disorders. To harness the human body's pain-reducing chemicals for use in treating medical disorders would solve a giant portion of the puzzle of pain.

Gate Control Theory

In 1965, Drs. Ronald Melzack and Patrick Wall* proposed a theory to explain how pain messages travel up the spinal cord to the brain. While the accuracy of this theory remains a topic of debate, there is little doubt that their theory, known as the Gate Control Theory, represents the single most important theoretical contribution to the field of pain research.

The gate theory suggests that a specialized group of nerve cells in the substantia gelatinosa (located in the butterfly-shaped portion of the spinal cord known as the dorsal horn) acts as a control mechanism similar to a valve or gate. The gate regulates the flow of pain messages into the central nervous system from peripheral nerves. When the gate is open, pain messages pass through to the brain and register pain. When the gate is closed, pain messages do not pass through and, theoretically, pain should not be experienced.

According to Drs. Melzack and Wall, small bundles of nerve fibre keep the gate open, and larger nerve-fibre bundles, whose messages travel faster than messages on the smaller bundles, can close the gate. Accordingly, if you pinch your finger in a desk drawer, the pain will slowly travel up small nerve-fibre bundles towards the brain. If you briskly rub your finger and hand, the response of rubbing will initiate a faster message along large nerve-fibre bundles, signalling the gate to close and limiting the amount of pain you experience.

*Dr. Melzack is a psychologist; Dr. Wall is a neuroanatomist.

Psychological variables also play a role in regulating the flow of pain messages through the gate. We may closely attend to the pain or use distraction techniques to keep our mind off pain. In addition, the expectation and stress of pain have an impact on the function of the gate.

PSYCHOLOGICAL MECHANISMS OF PAIN

Personality and Pain

Perhaps half of the distressing quality of chronic pain is psychological. This is not to say that half of all chronic-pain patients experience pain that is psychological in origin. Although pain that results from mental and emotional causes (psychogenic pain) is very real, it affects only a small portion of the patients who suffer chronic pain. A far more common occurrence is chronic pain that began with some physical injury or disorder.

When a victim is forced to deal with unrelenting pain for days, weeks, months and even years, the most stalwart and stable mind can falter. Chronic pain changes any sufferer's personality to some extent, and some individuals lose their ability to respond to their surroundings. We may concentrate less on interpersonal relationships than on the pain itself. Relationships then become troublesome rather than joyful. As the distress is prolonged over months, we may become withdrawn, moody, irritable and eventually depressed to the point where life's goals and responsibilities are forsaken.

Personality changes wrought by the persistence of pain are thought by some scientists to be rooted in anatomical connections between deep-seated pain reception centers in the thalamus of the brain and the frontal lobes of the cerebral hemispheres. The frontal lobes in general serve human conscious effort in directing day-to-day activities and planning long- and short-term events. The nerve centers of the frontal lobes must receive information from the environment surrounding the body, and the sensory nervous system supplies this information. Nerve fibre bundles then relay this information to areas of the brain where data from previous experiences is stored. Under ordinary circumstances, the process continues until a goal or set of goals is formulated. The brain motor systems then engage to carry out the planned process.

When new, incoming sensory information is experienced as painful, either because a pain message from a body part is received or because the sensory element is unpleasant as compared with prior experiences, the frontal lobe system of the brain becomes dominated by the incoming stimulus or stimuli. Our attention is then continuously diverted to the painful sensation. The painful stimulus is thought to interfere with our normal conscious thought processes. If a painful stimulus persists, a consistent, conscious effort and a great deal of mental energy are required to divert our attention away from the pain. If the pain is relatively mild, energy is easily replenished, and consciousness is easily directed as our will desires. However, when the painful stimulus is of high intensity, the psychological energy demands are great, fatigue sets in, and our conscious attention is drawn more and more to the painful problem.

This overview of how personality and mental processes become involved in the experience of chronic pain is an obvious oversimplification of brain mechanisms and the complex interplay of physical and psychological variables. Numerous other factors such as fear, distraction, anxiety, depression, expectations and stress play important roles in shaping our perception of pain and influencing our ability either to effectively live with chronic pain or be controlled and disabled by it.

Less independent individuals, for example, often desire to be cared for by those around them. Many times, however, a dependency role is not possible, as in the case of heads of families. If such individuals wish relief from their roles as supporters and leaders, a chronic-pain problem can satisfy a secret desire for dependence, without the embarrassment of an open admission. A mild pain is magnified or the symptoms of a cured disorder are prolonged. The patient, consciously or unconsciously, needs pain to satisfy long-standing emotional needs.

A similar situation can exist with chronic-pain victims whose premorbid personality (personality prior to the onset of pain) is marked by dissatisfaction and unhappiness. Perhaps discontent is the result of a boring career, advanced age, marital dissatisfaction or family role. To a person "trapped" in one of these unpleasant situations, even daily tasks become drudgery. Chronic pain may provide the excuse to cease performing burdensome tasks and, because of the sympathy of family and friends, the victim can still maintain a respected role in the eyes of others.

Expectations and Pain

A simple suspicion that has recently been verified experimentally is this: If you expect something to hurt, it probably will. Again, we emphasize the complex relationship between the mind and body. This relationship is so complex and the interplay of psychological and physical variables so confounded, that to fully explain or separate the mind from the body is an impossible task. Consider, for example, this 1889 medical report from Dr. C. Lloyd Tuckey, a physician.

> There are few cases of this kind more remarkable than one related by Mr. Woodhouse Braine, the well-known chloroformist. Having to administer ether to an hysterical girl who was about to be operated on for the removal of two sebaceous tumors from the scalp, he found that the ether bottle was empty, and that the inhalling bag was free from even the odor of any anesthetic. While a fresh supply was being obtained, he thought to familiarize the patient with the process by putting the inhaling bag over her mouth and nose, and telling her to breathe quietly and deeply. After a few inspirations, she cried, "Oh, I feel it; I am going off," and a moment after, her eyes turned up, and she became unconscious. As she was found to be perfectly insensible and the ether had not yet come, Mr. Braine proposed that the surgeon should proceed with the operation. One tumor was removed without in the least disturbing her, and then, in order to test her condition, a bystander said that she was coming to. Upon this she began to show signs of waking, so the bag was once more applied, with the remark, "She'll soon be off again," when she immediately lost sensation and the operation was successfully and painlessly completed.*

*Mastering Pain, p. 34.

Further substantiating the powerful influence of expectation in our experience is the phenomenon of placebo drugs. Placebos are usually plain salt or sugar pills with no active ingredients, yet the placebo effect on pain is often remarkable. Patients taking placebos are given the suggestion that they are powerful and effective drugs. For many pain patients, the expectation of relief produces pain relief that approaches the effectiveness of powerful analgesic drugs.

The role of pain intensity and expectation can also have an opposite effect. In one study, subjects were given two separate electrical shocks. Before each shock, subjects were given a description of what was to occur. The first description did not include the word "pain" or "painful," while the second description did. As you might guess, the second shock was consistently rated as more painful than the first even though the intensity of the electrical shocks was the same.

In cases of chronic pain, it is the chronic, never-ending nature of the disease that alters our expectations. The depression and frustration of living in constant distress can soon deplete our optimism and expectations for relief. In time, we come to expect pain, and as our expectation of pain increases, so too does our pain. It soon becomes a cycle—the more we hurt, the more we expect to hurt; the more we expect to hurt, the more we hurt, and so on. Breaking the cycle of pain and expectation requires a determined and consistent effort. Chapter Twelve will outline some hints to help you modify your attitude towards pain.

Stress and Pain

In recent years emotional stress has been linked to a variety of physical disorders. A sampling of some of these disorders includes bronchial asthma, cardiovascular disease, obesity, gastrointestinal disorders (such as peptic ulcers), tension headaches, dermatological disorders (such as neurodermatitis), and, of course, pain. The effects of stress on pain appear to be threefold. First, emotional stress can precipitate a physical disorder, such as muscle-contraction headaches (Chapters Three and Eight) and certain types of cardiovascular disorders. Second, stress can deplete your body of the "psychological energy" required to cope effectively with chronic pain on a daily basis. Third, emotional stress can intensify already existing pain since stress is associated with muscle tension, fatigue and pain.

Dr. Beverly J. Volicer recently reported an interesting investigation of the relationship between stress and pain.* The results of this study suggest that reducing hospital stress can result in less analgesic drug use, reduced hospital stay and less pain. Conversely, high stress and anxiety levels resulted in increased pain and more numerous difficulties with digestion, mood and sleep.

Throughout the remainder of this book, you will find a description of techniques to help you cope with stress and pain. Some of these techniques include physical exercise (Chapter Six), biofeedback (Chapter Seven), relaxation techniques (Chapter Ten) and cognitive pain management (Chapter Eleven). After reviewing these chapters, work hard towards getting into a "chronic pain management habit" by practicing some of these techniques daily. With practice, determination and the approval and help of your family doctor, you can learn to manage chronic pain!

---

*Beverly J. Volicer, Dr., "Hospital Stress and Patient Reports of Pain," *Journal of Human Stress*, June 1978, p. 28–37. Dr. Volicer is a psychiatrist.

CHAPTER THREE

Some Factors That May Cause Chronic Pain

Pain is the most common symptom of disease which compels us to seek medical counsel. Whereas acute symptomatic pain serves the useful purpose of warning us that something is wrong and is a useful diagnostic aid for physicians, in its chronic pathologic form, pain often imposes severe emotional, physical and economic stresses on the patient, his family and society.

Even more important than the billions of dollars spent yearly and the numerous workdays lost because of persistent pain is the cost of chronic distress in terms of human suffering. There are millions of suffering individuals who are not getting the relief from chronic pain that they deserve. Many of these individuals are exposed to a high risk of iatrogenic complications from improper medical treatment, including narcotic addiction, or are subjected to multiple, often useless, and at times mutilating, surgical procedures. A significant number understandably give up medical care and consult quacks. Quacks not only deplete the individual's financial resources, but often do harm: Some individuals with severe, intractable pain become so desperate that they commit suicide.

What is the cause of such devastating and persistent pain? Unfortunately, we do not know all of the causes of chronic pain. However, there seem to be several major sources of intractable pain that deserve particular attention.

MUSCLE PAIN

Muscular pain probably accounts for more health complaints in the United States than any other source of chronic pain. Most of us have experienced mild and temporary muscular pain and are greatly relieved when, several days later, we are back to our old selves again and feeling fine. But for some, the discomfort of muscular pain never ceases.

Back Pain

Back pain can have a variety of causes, including congenital postural abnormalities, trauma or injury to the back or neck (such as whiplash) or bad posture. A frequent source of chronic back pain can be linked to degenerative diseases of the intricate muscle and ligament structures in the skeleton that allow humans to walk upright. The fact that walking upright places a tremendous strain on the delicate supporting structures of the back and spine, combined with the frequency of back-pain complaints, has led some to wonder if humans were really ever intended to walk upright or whether our standard mode of locomotion is nothing more than an evolutionary mix-up! Dystrophy (weakening or degeneration) and disease often attack the back's muscle and discs, which act as cushions between a chain of blocks (the vertebrae) stacked one on the other. The muscles and discs are kept from collapsing by a marvelously exact system of muscles and ligaments that acts with magnificent synergistic and antagonistic precision. If these discs slip out of place or become crushed, back pain is usually inevitable.

Trauma is another common cause of back pain which most often affects the axial muscles in the small of the back or lumbar area. Thousands of people injure their backs daily because of injudicious lifting, a fall or an athletic injury. The main reason for the prevalence of these strain injuries is that so many people are in poor physical condition. Most muscle strains and back pain could be avoided by proper weight control, daily exercise to keep trim and retain good muscle tone, and a regular schedule of sports activities consistent with age and body physique.

Athletes and healthy young people seldom injure their backs because they are usually in excellent physical shape. However, most people over thirty years of age become physically sluggish, gain weight and exercise sporadically, if at all. When they do exercise, it is often a strenuous workout at an aggressive sport.

Low-back pain is also very common in women who have repeated pregnancies with excessive weight gain and who fail to recondition themselves with postpartum exercises. These women often develop a state of poor muscle tone, obesity and spinal deterioration that leads to chronic pain.

Tension, which can generate muscle spasms, is another major source of chronic muscle pain in the back. Low-back muscle spasms often start with strain or trauma to the region (incorrect lifting or accidents can cause such trauma) and are then further aggravated by worrying about the pain, or by any of life's stresses that accumulate in our daily activities.

Though low-back spasms are common, it is sometimes hard for doctors to find evidence that tension and spasms are causing the pain; the spasms may not be present at the time of a medical examination. If the doctor questions you about your life, you may answer that everything is great, not consciously realizing that you are under stress or tension, though you actually may be. Once spasmodic low-back pain is diagnosed, however, you will likely be told that the spasms caused by tension are reversible with the aid of physical therapy, exercise and/or biofeedback (Chapter Seven).

NEURAL PAIN

It comes as no surprise that the nerves are a key piece in the chronic-pain puzzle. After all, the nerves are responsible for picking up pain messages from different parts of the body and transmitting them to the brain and then back again to the site where the message began. The brain alone has billions of nerves and free nerve endings. Involvement or injury to a nerve may result in disorders such as neuralgia or neuritis. Neuralgia is nerve pain that feels like stabbing or severe throbbing along a nerve pathway. Neuritis is an inflammation of a nerve that may be caused by a viral infection, mechanical irritation or reduced blood flow. Neuritis feels like a deep burning pain, and the affected area may become highly sensitive or numb. Paralysis and muscle atrophy (wasting away) may also result in the area of the body supplied by the nerve.

Trigeminal Neuralgia

Nerves throughout the human body have been divided by scientists in such a way that the twelve major nerves whose function is primarily to the head and neck are collectively referred to as the cranial nerves. Of the cranial nerves, the trigeminal (fifth cranial nerve) is sometimes the culprit in cases of chronic facial pain. Trigeminal neuralgia, sometimes referred to as tic douloureux, is an irritation of the trigeminal nerve which is usually caused by either trauma to the nerve or by a viral infection. The deep stabbing neuralgia can be set off by as little as a puff of wind or the slightest touch against the face. The pain is usually intermittent, disappearing within a few hours, only to return again and again. In many cases, trigeminal neuralgia can be effectively treated with the anticonvulsive drug Tegretol®.

Postherpetic Neuralgia

Remember your bout with chicken pox when you were a child? Undoubtedly, the experience was unpleasant. An adult's confrontation with *herpes zoster*, the virus that causes chicken pox in children, is even more unpleasant and results in a condition called postherpetic neuralgia. The viral infection produces lesions on the skin that are similar to chicken pox marks. The major problem, however, involves the lesions produced under the skin on the nerve fibres of both the central and sympathetic nervous systems. Large nerve fibres may be destroyed, leaving a greater quantity of small nerve fibres, which act as transmitters of pain messages. The result is that pain messages are sent, and there are no corresponding nerves to countermand them with messages signalling relief. This condition is even further aggravated in older persons who have atherosclerosis (fatty deposits in the arteries that decrease the blood flow to parts of the body). There has been some experimentation with the drugs Elavil® (an antidepressant) and Prolixin® (an antipsychotic) to treat postherpetic neuralgia, but the results thus far are inconclusive.

Neuromas

When a nerve is crushed or injured in some way, the body releases a number of chemicals that assist in the repair or regeneration of the fibre. Unfortunately, most often the trauma destroys the channels through which the nerve should grow, so that sensory nerves, particularly small fibre pain nerves, become tangled into a mass, or tumor (neuroma). Neuromas can be extremely painful to the touch and result in a life of chronic pain. Some individuals seem more susceptible to developing neuromas than others. There appears to be no effective treatment for neuromas at the present time.

Palatal Myoclonus

This very rare syndrome is caused by damage to specific motor centers in the brain stem (the lower portion of the brain) which results in spasmodic muscular contractions in the soft palate, located at the upper-rear portion of the mouth. Other muscles in the head and neck may infrequently be involved, but usually the muscles in the roof of the mouth are the ones that involuntarily expand and contract rapidly in a rhythmic (myoclonic) motion. Palatal myoclonus can be caused by nerve damage that results from trauma, or it may be induced by a vascular disease near the brain stem. This is a rare syndrome whose etiology is often difficult to pinpoint. When the exact location of the disorder can be identified, surgery is occasionally effective.

Sympathetic Dystrophy

Intense chronic pain can be associated with a weakening or degeneration of sympathetic nerves. Sympathetic dystrophy is such a disorder and is usually caused by trauma that results in nerve damage. Individuals with sympathetic dystrophy complain of tingling, pin-and-needle sensations, and coldness in the affected area (usually a hand or foot). In extreme forms, hair loss and loss of bone from the fingertips or toetips is visible on X rays. This disorder can easily be detected with the use of thermography, which is a specialized test that detects temperature differences caused by cancer growth or by injuries to the nervous system or blood vessels. Using heat-sensitive detection devices, a photograph may be taken in which the damaged area shows up as either warmer (in cases of cancer) or colder (in cases of pain caused by damaged nerves or vessels) than the rest of the body. Sympathetic dystrophy is difficult to cure, although the repeated injection of a numbing substance in the area of the sympathetic nerves sometimes produces relief.

VASCULAR PAIN

The blood vessels act as conduits for blood flow throughout the human body. Vessels can be thought of as elastic tubing that are prone to constricting (vasoconstriction) and dilating (vasodilation) in response to numerous chemical and emotional stimuli. Vasoconstriction and vasodilation can produce a number of bodily responses, one being intense and chronic pain.

Migraine Headache

Migraine is a common disorder that interferes with normal life when it is severe and recurs frequently. It is essentially an episodic disorder in which blood is shunted away from the cerebral cortex and the scalp. As a result, the unfortunate sufferer may undergo a wide variety of symptoms. While the smaller vessels are constricted, the arteries dilate, giving rise to a headache that is commonly one-sided. The headache is usually accompanied by nausea, vomiting and sensitivity to light. The varied manifestations of migraine can be explained in terms of disordered control of blood vessels which overreact in response to emotional, physical and chemical stimuli. More will be said about migraine later in this chapter.

Atherosclerosis

Arteries damaged by the long-term buildup of yellowish-colored fatty deposits called plaques can also result in chronic pain. The buildup of these fatty deposits restricts the blood flow to parts of the body and is thought to be caused by a high cholesterol diet, although some individuals seem to have an inherited predisposition to developing this disorder.

Raynaud's Disease

Raynaud's disease is a disturbance of the cardiovascular system that leads to pale, cold hands or feet, pain, and the risk of gangrene in extreme cases. It is believed to be triggered by exposure to cold and/or stress. Raynaud's disease commonly has been treated with a surgical procedure known as sympathectomy: Nerves or nerve pathways in the area of the spinal cord are severed or cauterized by electrical current. More recently, other patients have been treated with vasodilator drugs in an effort to improve circulation to the affected limb. Unfortunately, most patients remain untreated because they have been told there is little that can be done for the disorder. The common suggestions are to keep the hands gloved and, if possible, to reside in a warm climate during the late fall and winter when the blanching and pain are most severe. Recently, biofeedback (Chapter Seven) has been used with some effectiveness in the treatment of this disorder.

TERMINAL DISEASE PAIN

Pain as a result of a terminal disease, such as cancer, greatly differs from other types of chronic pain. In the vast majority of chronic-pain states, the pain may continue for months, years or a lifetime. Also, the pain of a terminal disease is most often easily identified, whereas the etiology of many chronic-pain states remains a mystery.

Cancer

Terminal cancer has both a primary and secondary cause for the intense pain that is associated with some forms of the disease. The primary cause is blockage of organs by tumor growth that displaces organs from their intended position in the body. Therefore, pain can result from the gradual destruction of organs, bones and other tissue by tumors, and also from a direct attack by cancer growth on the nerves. There are a number of secondary sources of terminal cancer pain. First, radiation, which is sometimes used to treat certain types of cancer, may produce scarring that traps nerves and produces pain. Second, chemotherapy, also used to treat certain types of cancer, frequently causes severe and repeated nausea. Third, many cancer patients must submit to repeated bone marrow sampling and blood sampling. The taking of bone marrow samples is often quite painful, while repeated puncture of the veins can cause inflammation, after which subsequent attempts to draw samples or to start intravenous infusions can be very painful. Finally, the gravity of a terminal disease produces heightened emotional anguish and anxiety which results in both psychic pain and intensified physical discomfort.

PHANTOM LIMB PAIN

Phantom limb pain can result following the amputation of a limb and represents a very bizarre and fascinating disorder. Patients report feeling a severe and unrelenting pain in their foot, leg or arm, even though the limb has been amputated. Phantom limb pain is thought to result from the destruction of nerve endings in the amputated part of the body. Transcutaneous electrical nerve stimulation (Chapter Six) and hypnosis (Chapter Eight) are frequently used to treat this disorder.

GASTROINTESTINAL PAIN

Colitis, chronic constipation, hemorrhoids, gallstones, pancreatitis, ileitis, polyps, ulcers and heartburn are all sources of chronic intestinal and stomach pain. Some of these disorders, such as ileitis, ulcers, colitis and heartburn, are intensified by anxiety and emotional stress. In fact, peptic ulcers are sometimes referred to as "the executive's disease" because of the important role played by anxiety and stress in the overall disease process. Other gastrointestinal disorders are thought to be associated with degenerative diseases caused by impairment of a major organ such as the gallbladder or liver.

There seems to be a number of contributing factors involved in gastrointestinal pain. Overdoses of laxatives and improper diet can cause chronic constipation and/or stomachache. Overindulgence in alcohol can bring on pancreatitis and gastritis (an irritation of the stomach lining). Ingestion of excessive amounts of aspirin for whatever reason, including headaches caused by the overindulgence of alcohol, can also lead to gastritis. Too much coffee or any other beverage containing caffeine can contribute to diarrhea and eventual gastritis. Chronic alcohol abuse can really damage the stomach lining and cause cirrhosis of the liver. Anxiety, frustration, tension and emotional stress can aggravate any of these disorders.

JOINT PAIN

The human skeletal system is a highly complex and remarkable supportive structure. It is strong enough to allow us to stand upright, yet it is designed in such a way as to allow us to bend, stoop, walk and run. We can move about freely because of numerous joints throughout the body where bones connect, similar to hinges on a door. Unfortunately, because of a number of factors, joints are also susceptible to injury and disease which can result in chronic pain.

Arthritis

The most common form of joint pain is arthritis. There are several forms of arthritis, including rheumatoid, osteo and gonorrheal; however, any inflammation of a joint is known as arthritis. The pain of arthritis can be due directly to the swelling of the joint that exerts pressure on the ligaments and other soft tissues surrounding the joints. Pain can also result from stiffness due to swelling that limits the use of the joint, which in turn promotes further stiffness and pain.

Rheumatoid Arthritis

Rheumatoid arthritis is a virulent form of arthritis that causes the soft tissue and skin surrounding the affected joints to thicken into deformities. These changes in the muscles and connective tissues (ligaments) are thought to be caused by deposits of lymphocytes (cells from the lymph glands) that thicken the connective tissue. Lymphocytes normally are filtered out of the blood, but this process stops when arthritis sets in.

Gout

Gout, once referred to as the rich man's penance for his life-style of idleness and excessive food, now is known to be neither the exclusive preserve of the upper classes, nor the result of eating rich food. Gout is a buildup of uric acid in the joints. The acid is manufactured by the kidneys, and when the kidneys are impaired, they incorrectly process the acid so it is not eliminated through the urine. This malfunction can be controlled with a drug-therapy regimen and dietary adjustments.

HEADACHES

The most prevalent of all human diseases, headaches strike almost 90 percent of the world's population at least once a month. Over 15 million people in the United States are thought to suffer from migraine, the most painful of all headaches, while millions more are afflicted with chronic "tension" or muscle-contraction headaches.

Muscle-Contraction (Tension) Headaches

Over 90 percent of the people who suffer chronic headaches need never have them. They are not ill, and they have no special physical predisposition. On the surface there is nothing wrong with them, yet they suffer constantly. Their pain is real and excruciating, and is described in graphic terms as being like a tight band being wound around the forehead or a hammer beating inside the skull. Why is it that these people, over 25 million in the United States at a conservative count, are plagued in this manner? The answer is found in one deceptively simple word: tension.

Psychologically, the idea of tension is very complex, encompassing many different emotional states. But physiologically, it is easy to understand. The muscles are tense when they are prepared to take some action. To visualize this, you have only to flex the muscles in your arms or legs. This is their state during any physical exertion. If you keep the muscles in a state of tension without doing anything, you will soon begin to feel uncomfortable and will have to relax them after a while.

The mechanism of all tension headaches is a contraction of the muscles at the back of the head and neck above the shoulders. The tensed muscles impinge upon the nerves that travel up the spinal column into the brain. The contraction also squeezes the blood vessels, following essentially the same path. This constriction of the blood vessels and irritation of the nerves lead to a headache. The action of the "headache muscles" is involuntary, but the act of contraction occurs for exactly the same reason that all the other muscles tense and relax. The headache muscles have gotten their signals crossed: They have been misled into anticipating an act of physical exertion and have needlessly prepared for it. Muscles can be said to "think," in that they often act independently of instructions from the brain. But they may not always think well: They may confuse neural messages, tensing at the wrong moment and maintaining tension when there is no reason to do so.

The brain is an organ that has continually evolved with the development of the species—it did not exist in its present form in the first human creature. The thoughts and actions of early man were controlled from a point now known as the old brain. The primitives led a very simple mental and emotional life. Their movements were dictated by elemental instincts and reflexes. Anthropologists believe that the stiffening of the head and neck muscles was a protective reaction from either an attack or a torrential forest downpour. It was an expression of fright; the body was preparing to defend itself. Today we also hunch our shoulders when caught in a rainstorm, although this gesture serves no purpose. Like a turtle retreating into its shell, we try to keep the hostile environment at bay.

What started as a reaction to immediate danger became a standard reflex withdrawal from all unpleasantness. As civilization became more complex, the stark terror of primeval man was replaced by a subtler type of fear known as anxiety. Where the primitives must have spent most of their lives cringing from the unknown, contemporary man knows very few moments of abject fear. We may go a whole lifetime without being afraid for our lives or facing any physical menace whatsoever. But very few of us can last a day without having at least one moment of anxiety.

The categories of anxiety are too numerous to detail. But in many people the body's reaction to all of them is the same: The "headache muscles" tighten up and remain tightened. Anxiety does not have the immediate quality of fear. It does not come and go quickly, but lingers on, giving the rest of the body plenty of time to react. It increases the secretion of certain hormones, some of which have an effect on the blood vessels. Adrenaline, the "fight or flight" hormone released when there is great stress or danger, also dribbles out in times of anxiety. The body acts as if it were in danger. There seems to be no communication between the primitive protective reflex and the part of the consciousness that deals with reality.

Aspirin is most often taken for tension headaches. Its active chemical is acetylsalicylic acid, which was originally derived from the bark of the willow tree. First used in the 1760's, it was put into commercial form by the Bayer Aspirin Company of Germany in 1899. Aspirin is now the most popular medication in the world. The consumption of aspirin in the United States alone is estimated at 20 billion tablets a year.* Recently, biofeedback (Chapter Seven) has shown excellent results in treating chronic muscle-contraction headaches.

Migraine Headaches

About one out of every ten Americans suffers from migraine or vascular headaches. Though they affect fewer people than tension headaches do, migraines can be far more severe, disabling and difficult to treat.

Migraines are characterized by intense pain, usually located on one side of the head, and by a distinct throbbing

---

*George Peterfy, "Hypnosis," *Psychosomatic Medicine*, Ed Wittkower and H. Warnes, eds. (Hagerstown, Maryland: Harper & Row, 1977), p. 130.

sensation in the temples, like a pulse. The victim may experience nausea, changes in vision (such as spots or geometric shapes in front of the eyes), temporary loss of vision, double vision, or sharply increased sensitivity to light just before and during a migraine attack.

Migraines tend to recur at regular intervals: Most migraine victims can tell when an attack is imminent. Headaches may last for only a few hours, or for as long as two or three days. They may be so intense as to virtually incapacitate the victims, forcing the sufferer to do nothing but stay in bed in a quiet, darkened room. Many migraine victims report distinct mood changes just before and occasionally after a migraine attack, ranging from depression, irritability and confusion to elation and euphoria. Some report feeling a numbness in the opposite side of the body from the side of the head that hurts.

Researchers consider the causes of migraine to involve complex cycles of change in the body's vascular system. Factors such as sleep patterns, stress, genetic predisposition, hormone levels, allergies, weather patterns, fluid intake, and even ingredients in such common foods as chocolate, bananas, nuts, pork, red wine and certain cheeses have been implicated in the onset of certain types of migraine.

A number of drugs that work by constricting the blood vessels, especially ergotamine tartrate and methysergide maleate, are used to treat migraine, but they can have adverse side effects and can be addictive. Surgical procedures for alleviating severe migraine pain were attempted during the Forties and Fifties but were found ineffective.

Experiments have shown that specific complex patterns of change in the circulation of blood in the head characterize the onset of migraine. The arteries constrict, then dilate. There are related biochemical changes, and there is a general increase in activity of the sympathetic nervous system. This knowledge forms the theoretical framework for the current application of thermal biofeedback (Chapter Seven) in the treatment of migraine headaches.

Cluster Headaches (Migrainous Neuralgia)

Cluster headache is the only type of headache that primarily strikes men: Some 85 percent of all those affected by this type of headache are males. A curious intermittent pattern of bouts or clusters of intensely severe pains which recur once, twice or even up to ten times in 24 hours (which can continue for weeks or months) are symptoms of cluster headaches. The pain then disappears in eight out of ten victims and goes into recess for months or years. It then comes back with its previous intensity for another devastating bout. The condition is often confused with trigeminal neuralgia because of the severity of the pain, but unlike trigeminal neuralgia, which strikes with stabs as brief as a lightning flash, the pains in cluster headache last from ten minutes to several hours at a time. It is also confused with migraine, hence the alternative term "migrainous neuralgia," which is still preferred in Great Britain. But only in about 20 percent of all patients do the pains recur regularly, without intermission, in the manner of migraine.

Cluster headaches are thought to be an allergic reaction, since histamine is found in the tissue cells on the affected side. Histamine (a substance that causes capillaries and veins to dilate) is released when there is an injury to the skin or membranes, such as a reaction by the membranes to an allergen. Recent experimentation suggests Lithium® (a drug frequently used to treat manic depression) is a useful treatment for selected victims of cluster headache.

Ice-Cream Headaches

Holding ice or ice cream in the mouth or swallowing it while it is still very cold may cause a localized pain in the palate or throat. A headache in the forehead or temple because of referred pain from the trigeminal nerve endings may sometimes occur. Occasionally it may produce pain behind the ear because this area is supplied by another cranial nerve, the glossopharyngeal, which also has branches over the back of the throat that may be thrown into sudden activity by intense cold. The cause of ice-cream headache is sudden cooling of the roof of the mouth. Cooling of the esophagus (the tube which connects the throat with the stomach) or the stomach itself does not cause the pain. Obviously, the cure for ice-cream headache is either to avoid eating ice cream or to ingest intensely cold substances at a slow and easy rate.

CHAPTER FOUR

Do You Have Chronic Pain?

Patients who suffer chronic pain have long presented a diagnostic enigma. Pain is a subjective symptom, and attempts to measure discomfort objectively have proven inadequate. Physical examinations and the use of standard diagnostic tests such as nerve conduction studies, myelograms, electromyography and X rays can often document an organic basis for chronic pain such as a lesion, traumatized or degenerative disc, muscular impairment and joint inflammation. While these tests serve a very useful purpose and are fine as far as they go, standard diagnostic techniques suffer three major problems. First, they are inexact and frequently do not provide accurate information. Second, the absence of positive findings on a myelogram or other objective test does not mean that the patient is not in pain. Some pain syndromes defy definition by available medical testing. Third, standard diagnostic tests do not take into account that chronic pain is a disease in itself.

Most of us are at least vaguely familiar with X rays, nerve conduction studies (the ability of a nerve to conduct impulses properly), myelograms (essentially X rays of the spinal cord following injection of a radiopaque medium), and electromyography (graphic recording of muscle activity following electrical stimulation). Two newer diagnostic techniques, thermography and the computed tomographic scanner, are currently gaining popularity in the evaluation of chronic-pain states.

Thermography has long been used as a technique to diagnose abnormalities of the female breast, including cancer, but it has only recently been employed in the physical diagnosis of pain states. If pain is the result of restricted blood flow to some part of the body, thermography will record a thermal picture of the affected part, showing the blood-restricted area as "cooler" than surrounding heat-producing tissue. Thermography has proven most effective in the diagnosis of pain resulting from trauma or damage to the sympathetic nerves.

The newest physical diagnostic technique used in the evaluation of pain is the computed tomographic scanner, better known as the CAT scanner or CT scanner. The CT scanner combines computers, X rays and photographic film to produce cross-sectional views of all body parts including the brain. Viewing cross sections is similar to looking at the individual slices of a loaf of bread. The CT scanner can identify lesions that are difficult or impossible for X rays to detect.

Highly sophisticated technological advances are extremely important in the diagnosis of chronic pain, but they address only the physical component. Since many psychological variables naturally enter into a patient's interpretation of and response to chronic pain, psychological testing has increasingly become utilized as an adjunct to physical diagnostic procedures. If your physician requests that you see a clinical psychologist for testing, do not be alarmed. Rather than thinking you are "crazy" or that your pain is "all in your head," your physician is simply attempting to provide the most comprehensive diagnostic workup possible of your pain. Psychological testing provides information in the same way that myelograms, X rays, nerve conduction studies and electromyography provide information. Chronic pain has both physical and psychological components, and only with the availability of all relevant information can your physician most accurately diagnose your discomfort and best provide for your treatment.

The most widely used psychological test in the evaluation of chronic pain is the Minnesota Multiphasic Personality Inventory, better known as the MMPI. This inventory is a 400- or 566-item test (depending on the form used), consisting of true/false answers to a wide variety of questions. The patient's responses to questions are tabulated in a profile which is interpreted by a clinical psychologist in much the same manner that an X ray is interpreted by a radiologist or other physician. Various personality traits are identified by the MMPI which can provide useful information, such as the role of psychological variables in a patient's pain complaints, which patients are most likely to benefit from surgery, the degree of depression and/or anxiety that the patient is experiencing as a result of his pain, and much more. As more and more physicians learn the value of psychological testing as an adjunct to physical diagnostic procedures, the use of psychological evaluations is becoming increasingly popular and accepted as a routine part of a comprehensive diagnostic procedure.

In 1977, Dr. Nelson Hendler and his colleagues at Johns Hopkins Hospital, Baltimore, Maryland, designed a screening test that is specifically for chronic back-pain patients.* Questions were formulated after conducting psychological evaluations on over 600 patients treated at a chronic-pain treatment center. The test was formulated and refined on the basis of how these different groups of patients responded to a series of questions regarding their pain experience and history, and significant related matters such as work, sexual activity, use of medications and thoughts of suicide. Depending on each patient's score, he or she will fall into one of the three diagnostic categories which follow:

A. TYPE I. This category describes individuals who show a normal response to chronic pain. If indicated, the patient will probably respond well to surgery and is usually willing to participate in all modalities of therapy, including exercise and psychotherapy.

B. TYPE II. This category describes individuals who may be considered "exaggerating pain patients." Surgery or other intervention procedures may be recommended with caution since many Type II patients do not respond well to surgery. Type II patients have found a use for chronic pain. The most effective mode of treatment is from a chronic-pain center with an emphasis on attitude change towards the pain.

C. TYPE III. This category describes individuals who should

*N. Hendler, M. Viernstein, P. Gucer and D. Long, "A Preoperative Screening Test for Chronic Back-Pain Patients," *Psychosomatics*, 1979, p. 20, 801–808.

receive care from a clinical psychologist or psychiatrist. This category describes the type of personality that freely admits to a great many pre-pain problems and shows considerable difficulty coping with the chronic pain they now experience. Surgery or other intervention should not be carried out without prior approval of a psychological/psychiatric consultation.

If you're interested in knowing how your chronic pain affects you and how you handle your pain, spend about ten minutes to complete the following screening test. You should remember that the following test is designed to screen patients for appropriate treatment decisions and is only one of many components involved in making a diagnosis. Do not take the results of this test out of context! It is presented only for your interest.

Hendler 10-Minute Screening Test
For Chronic Back Pain Patients

INSTRUCTIONS
The following test should take you about ten minutes to complete. For each question choose the statement that most closely applies to you, and mark down the number of points you receive on a separate sheet of paper. This test is specifically designed for back-pain patients and may not accurately reflect responses to other types of pain.

I. How did the pain that you now experience occur?
   (a) Sudden onset with accident or definable event _____ 0
   (b) Slow, progressive onset without acute exacerbation ____ 1
   (c) Slow, progressive onset with acute exacerbation without accident or event _____ 2
   (d) Sudden onset without an accident or definable event __ 3

II. Where do you experience the pain?
   (a) One site, specific, well-defined, consistent with anatomical distribution _____ 0
   (b) More than one site, each well-defined and consistent with anatomical distribution _____ 1
   (c) One site, inconsistent with anatomical considerations, or not well-defined _____ 2
   (d) Vague description, more than one site, of which one is inconsistent with anatomical considerations, or not well-defined or anatomically explainable _____ 3

---

*Test copyright 1979 by Nelson Hendler, M.D., M. S. Reprinted by permission.

III. Do you ever have trouble falling asleep at night or are you ever awakened from sleep?

(If the answer is "no", score 3 points and go to question IV. If the answer is "yes" proceed:)

IIIA. What keeps you from falling asleep, or what awakens you from sleep?
- (a) Trouble falling asleep every night due to pain _____ 0
- (b) Trouble falling asleep due to pain more than three times a week _____ 1
- (c) Trouble falling asleep due to pain less than three times per week _____ 2
- (d) No trouble falling asleep due to pain _____ 3
- (e) Trouble falling asleep which is not related to pain _____ 4

IIIB.
- (a) Awakened by pain every night _____ 0
- (b) Awakened from sleep by pain more than three times a week _____ 1
- (c) Not awakened from sleep by pain more than twice a week _____ 2
- (d) Not awakened from sleep by pain _____ 3
- (e) Restless sleep, or early morning awakening with or without being able to return to sleep, both unrelated to pain _ 4

IV. Does weather have any effect on your pain?
- (a) The pain is always worse in both cold and damp weather _ 0
- (b) The pain is always worse with damp weather or with cold weather _____ 1
- (c) The pain is occasionally worse with cold or damp weather _____ 2
- (d) The weather has no effect on the pain _____ 3

V. How would you describe the type of pain that you have?
- (a) Burning; or sharp, shooting pain; or pins and needles; or coldness; or numbness _____ 0
- (b) Dull, aching pain, with occasional sharp shooting pains not helped by heat _____ 1
- (c) Spasm-type pain, tension-type pain, or numbness over the area, relieved by massage or heat _____ 2
- (d) Nagging or bothersome pain _____ 3
- (e) Excruciating, overwhelming, or unbearable pain, relieved by massage or heat _____ 4

VI. How frequently do you have pain?
- (a) The pain is constant _____ 0

(b) The pain is nearly constant, occurring 50%–80% of the time _____ 1

(c) The pain is intermittent, occurring 25%–50% of the time _ 2

(d) The pain is only occasionally present, occurring less than 25% of the time _____ 3

VII. What medications have you used in the past month?

(a) No medications at all _____ 0

(b) Use of non-narcotic pain relievers or mild tranquillizers or antidepressants _____ 1

(c) Less than three-times-a-week use of a narcotic, sleeping pill, or tranquillizer _____ 2

(d) Greater than four-times-a-week use of narcotic, sleeping pill, or tranquillizer _____ 3

VIII. Does movement or position have any effect on the pain?

(a) The pain is unrelieved by position change or rest, and there have been previous operations for the pain _____ 0

(b) The pain is worsened by use, standing, or walking; and is relieved by lying down or resting the part _____ 1

(c) Position change and use have variable effects on the pain_ 2

(d) The pain is not altered by use or position change, and there have been no previous operations for the pain __ 3

IX. What hobbies do you have, and can you still participate in them?

(a) Unable to participate in any hobbies that were formerly enjoyed _____ 0

(b) Reduced number of hobbies or activities relating to a hobby _____ 1

(c) Still able to participate in hobbies but with some discomfort _____ 2

(d) Participate in hobbies as before _____ 3

X. How frequently did you have sex and orgasms before the pain, and how frequently do you have sex and orgasms now?

(a1) Sexual contact, prior to pain, three to four times a week, with no difficulty with orgasm; now sexual contact is 50% or less than previously, and coitus is interrupted by pain _____ 0

(a2) (For people over 45) Sexual contact twice a week with a 50% reduction in frequency since the pain _____ 0

(a3) (For people over 65) Sexual contact once a week, with a 50% reduction in frequency of coitus since the onset of pain _____ 0

(b) Pre-pain adjustment as defined above (a1-a3) with no difficulty with orgasm; now loss of interest in sex and/or difficulty with orgasm or erection _____ 1

(c) No change in sexual activity now as opposed to before the onset of pain _____ 2

(d) Unable to have sexual contact since the onset of pain, and difficulty with orgasm or erection *prior* to the pain _ 3

(e) No sexual contact prior to the pain, or absence of orgasm *prior* to the pain _____ 4

XI. Are you still working or doing your household chores?

(a) Working every day at the same pre-pain job or same level of household duties _____ 0

(b) Working every day but the job is not the same as pre-pain job, with reduced responsibility or physical activity ____ 1

(c) Working sporadically or doing a reduced amount of household chores _____ 2

(d) Not working at all or all household chores are now performed by others _____ 3

XII. What is your income now compared with before your injury or the onset of pain, and what are your sources of income?

(a) Any one of the following answers scores _____ 0
   1. Experiencing financial difficulty with family income 50% or less than previously
   2. Was retired and is still retired
   3. Patient is still working and is not having financial difficulties

(b) Experiencing financial difficulty with family income only 50%–75% of the pre-pain income _____ 1

(c) Patient unable to work, and receives some compensation so that the family income is at least 75% of the pre-pain income _____ 2

(d) Patient unable to work and receives no compensation but the spouse works and family income is still 75% of the pre-pain income _____ 3

(e) Patient doesn't work, yet the income from disability or other compensation sources is 80% or more of gross pay before the pain; the spouse does not work _____ 4

XIII. Are you suing anyone, or is anyone suing you, or do you have an attorney helping you with compensation or disability payments?

(a) No suit pending, and do not have an attorney _____ 0

(b) Litigation is pending, but is not related to the pain _____ 1

   (c) The patient is being sued as the result of an accident ___ 2
   (d) Litigation is pending or workmen's compensation case
      with a lawyer _____ 3 ✓

XIV. If you had three wishes for anything in the world, what
     would you wish for?
   (a) "Get rid of the pain" is the only wish _____ 0 ✓
   (b) "Get rid of the pain" is one of the three wishes _____ 1
   (c) My wishes would be something of a personal nature,
      such as having more money, having a better relationship
      with my spouse, or having a bigger house _____ 2
   (d) My wishes would be for something like peace in the
      world, an end to hunger, or something else for others _ 3

XV. Have you ever been depressed or thought of suicide?
   (a) I have been depressed, or I have been depressed in addi-
      tion to my pain, my depression makes me cry at times or
      think of suicide _____ 0 ✓
   (b) Because of the pain, I have been depressed, and I've felt
      guilty and angry _____ 1
   (c) I felt depressed before the pain, or before the pain I
      suffered a financial or personal loss (death of a friend,
      family member moved away), and now with the pain
      here, I also have some depression _____ 2
   (d) I don't feel depressed, I don't have crying jags, or I don't
      feel blue _____ 3
   (e) Before the pain I had a history of suicide attempts ____ 4

POINT TOTAL

Now add all your points and turn back to the description of the
three types of pain categories to see how personality variables may
be influencing your pain. A score of 18 points or less suggests that
you are a Type I personality; 19 to 31 points, Type II personality; and
32 or more points, Type III personality.

REMEMBER: This screening device is but one of many techniques,
both physical and psychological, that your doctor may use in
evaluating your pain. Taken alone, it has little value other than being
of interest.

17 points

CHAPTER FIVE

Drug Treatment of Chronic Pain

Drugs are without question the most commonly used pain-relief method employed today. In fact, drugs employed for the relief of pain are the most widely used of *all* pharmacological classes and are of undeniable importance to man. This is not without good reason: They are easy to administer, are relatively inexpensive and their effects are usually predictable. Drug treatment of pain is today a physician's first line of treatment which works for many pain patients. For others, unfortunately, drugs serve to multiply the many problems of pain.

A major problem with the use of drugs in the treatment of chronic pain is that medicines proven effective in the relief of acute pain are often ineffective and even harmful when used to treat chronic pain. For acute, temporary pain disorders, the potential adverse side effects of powerful analgesic drugs (drugs used to decrease pain) are overshadowed by the urgent need to relieve the patient's suffering. For instance, there is little hesitancy about administering a powerful painkilling drug to a patient who has just suffered a severe second-degree burn over 30 percent of his body. Nor is it reasonable to worry about the patient becoming dependent on the drug in such a critical case. Though it may be urgent, the need for pain relief is temporary, and a physician runs little risk of causing chemical dependence in a drug-treatment program that may last a week or two.

Recently, doctors have become increasingly aware that analgesic drug use in the treatment of acute pain is beneficial, while it can prove to be disastrous in the treatment of chronic pain. Powerful painkillers can cause serious toxic side effects when used in high doses for extended periods and can also cause severe psychological and physical dependence. In addition, there is now substantial evidence that powerful analgesic drugs lose their effectiveness in reducing pain after four to six weeks of administration. Many doctors have looked on in frustration as their patient's chronic pain continued untouched while their addiction grew steadily stronger.

Since describing several hundred different types of drugs which can be used in the treatment of pain is far beyond the scope of this book, three general classes of frequently used medication will be discussed: narcotic analgesics, nonnarcotic analgesics and psychotropic drugs. The general overview to follow is intended for informational purposes only. Your doctor should approve and prescribe any drug that you take.

Narcotic Analgesics

Most narcotics are opiates; that is, derived from opium, a product of the poppy plant, *papaver somniferum*. The unripe seed capsules are incised and the exudate collected, dried and powdered. Opium powder contains many alkaloids such as heroin and methadone, but only morphine, codeine and papaverine are generally considered to be medically useful. Morphine and codeine are primarily used as analgesics, and papaverine serves as a smooth-muscle relaxant (antispasmodic).

In the past fifty years or so, a number of synthetic derivatives made by modification of the morphine molecule have been manufactured. These derivatives are termed opioids and include, among others, Dilaudid® (hydromorphone), Numorphan® (oxymorphone), Demerol® (meperidine) and Dolophine® (methadone). These structurally diverse compounds all share with morphine the ability to produce analgesia, respiratory depression, gastrointestinal spasm and physical dependence. None, however, has yet been demonstrated as significantly different from or superior to the prototypical narcotic analgesic morphine with respect to their important pharmacology. Morphine, consequently, will be considered the representative of the class narcotic analgesics.

Morphine and its congeners (synthetically derived compounds) primarily exert their effects on the smooth muscles of the gastrointestinal tract and the central nervous system. Indeed, the use of opium (which contains approximately ten percent morphine) for relief of diarrhea and dysentery preceded by centuries its use as an analgesic. The effects of morphine on the central nervous system are expressed as a combination of stimulation and depression, and include analgesia, drowsiness, respiratory depression and depression of the cough reflex.

Morphine-induced analgesia occurs without loss of consciousness and provides only symptomatic relief, without removing or altering the cause of pain. In therapeutic doses, there is a tranquillization or mood of calm and a drowsiness from which the patient is easily aroused. Subjective effects of morphine and its congeners appear to be dose-related. As the dose is increased, drowsiness becomes more pronounced and sleep ensues; the mood of peace and calm will also be accentuated with increased doses. The analgesic effect of narcotic "painkillers" is also enhanced as the dose is increased so that pain of a more severe nature will be relieved. Unfortunately, as the dose is increased, so too is the incidence of nausea and vomiting and the threats of respiratory depression (decreased or "shallow" breathing or even the cessation of breathing on overdose).

Exactly how morphine and its congeners induce analgesia is not completely understood at present. Many researchers believe that narcotics produce relief through chemical interactions within central nervous-system mechanisms, primarily those of the brain. Opiates interact with receptors, most of which are located in the limbic system of the brain, which in humans is primarily associated with the arousal of emotions. Rather than altering the peripheral chemical interaction or sensations that are responsible for sending pain messages to the brain, it is believed that narcotics work by changing the affective component of the pain experience. For example, after administration of a narcotic analgesic, a patient may report that the pain continues, but that it is no longer discomforting (that the pain can be tolerated with calm or indifference).

One of the more serious drawbacks of narcotic analgesic use is the threat of tolerance and physical dependence. Tolerance is defined as a decreased responsiveness to any drug as the result of prior administrations of the drug. More simply stated, after taking a narcotic drug for a period of time, the human body adapts and the drug loses some of its effectiveness. Consequently, increasingly larger doses must be administered to produce a level of pain relief equivalent to that of the initial administration.

Physical dependence refers to an abnormal physiological state produced by repeated administration of a drug (in this instance a narcotic), which then makes necessary the continued use of the drug to prevent the appearance of a withdrawal or abstinence syndrome. This threat is particularly meaningful to the chronic-pain patient who suffers months or years of discomfort and frequently searches for stronger and stronger drugs to "kill the pain." A major goal of many chronic-pain treatment centers is to withdraw the pain sufferer gradually from a physical dependence on narcotic analgesic drugs.

Despite the adverse side effects noted, morphine is a relatively safe drug when prescribed by a knowledgeable physician and remains the standard drug of choice in the treatment of many acute and severe pain states such as postoperative pain, multiple trauma and the acute pain of myocardial infarction. However, narcotic drugs have few if any appropriate uses in the treatment of chronic pain. As doctors become increasingly aware of the contraindications of narcotic use in intractable pain, many experts in the field of pain management expect the use and abuse of morphine and its congeners in the treatment of chronic-pain states to decrease substantially.

Codeine, like morphine and aspirin, is a naturally occurring substance and is frequently used to treat moderate to severe pain. Also like morphine and other opiates, codeine can cause adverse side effects, including depressed respiration, nausea and vomiting, dizziness and constipation. It is not nearly as addictive as morphine, but prolonged use of codeine can easily lead to increased tolerance.

Demerol® (meperidine) is a wholly synthetic analgesic and sedative supposedly free of many of morphine's undesirable side effects. In fact, Demerol® does not significantly differ from morphine in its important pharmacology. In therapeutic doses, it produces analgesia, sedation and respiratory depression, as well as other central nervous-system actions mentioned above as common to other narcotic analgesics. Regarding its supposed lack of undesirable properties, Demerol® is the narcotic most commonly abused by health professionals who still mistakenly believe that Demerol® has a lower threat of causing physical dependence and is easier to stop using than morphine. In fact, Demerol® abuse and dependence have been widely documented since the drug was first introduced, and it is now recognized that Demerol® differs little from morphine with respect to its potential for abuse and dependence.

Darvon® (propoxyphene) is also a wholly synthetic agent that is often used with patients who cannot tolerate codeine. At present, Darvon® is legally classified as a "nonnarcotic" and is usually prescribed as an analgesic for mild to moderate pain. Its legal status notwithstanding, Darvon® is classified under narcotic analgesics in this chapter because it is subject to abuse. Physical dependence can also develop during high-dose chronic use. In fact, there is no great difference between the dependence liabilities of codeine and Darvon®.

Nonnarcotic Analgesics

Drugs classified as nonnarcotic analgesics comprise a large, structurally heterogeneous group of compounds far too extensive to address adequately within the limitations of this chapter. Therefore, only selected drugs (those that are widely used and those with potentially unique application in pain states) will be discussed.

Aspirin (acetylsalicylic acid) is the most effective and important of the analgesics classified as nonnarcotics and, moreover, is the single most widely used drug in the world—narcotic and nonnarcotic alike. Because aspirin is a nonprescription drug and so readily available, it is generally not credited with the analgesic efficacy it in fact possesses. It is a very effective and useful analgesic in the relief of mild to moderate pain. In addition, when compared to other analgesics, aspirin is inexpensive and has a relatively low incidence of adverse side effects.

Aspirin and other nonnarcotic analgesics appear to reduce pain by interfering with the biochemistry of pain formation at peripheral nerve sites in the body. Unlike narcotic analgesics, aspirin does not alter the response to pain in the central nervous system and, therefore, has a lower analgesic effect. For example, 650 mg of aspirin is generally thought to produce relief from pain equivalent to 65 mg of codeine or Darvon®. Doses of aspirin exceeding 650 mg, however, do not increase peak analgesia (although the duration of effect may be prolonged), whereas increased doses of codeine, for instance, will provide greater relief from pain. Aspirin, it seems, has a "ceiling effect" around 650 mg, and doses beyond that amount do little to increase its effectiveness. Aspirin may have some slight effects on central nervous-system activity, but they are negligible when compared to those of morphine and other narcotic analgesics.

Although aspirin is relatively safe, does not cause physical dependence and is readily available, there is no such thing as a totally and completely safe drug. Overmedication can cause aspirin toxicity, which can be fatal. The symptoms of aspirin toxicity include hyperthermia (loss of body heat), cardiac arrhythmia (irregular heartbeat), shallow breathing, coma and even death. Fortunately, most cases of aspirin intoxication are not life-threatening when treated properly.

Acetaminophen (Tylenol®, Datril®, Tempra®, Liquiprin® and others) is approximately equal in analgesic strength to aspirin and has a mode of action in the body that is also similar to aspirin. Acetaminophen has enjoyed a surge of popularity in recent years, largely because it does not cause the minor gastric irritation and bleeding that aspirin can cause. For individuals allergic to aspirin or who suffer disorders in which aspirin is contraindicated (e.g., peptic ulcers), acetaminophen provides an effective aspirin substitute.

Psychotropic Drugs

An important third category of drugs is collectively termed psychotropic and has been recognized only recently as often effective in the treatment of chronic-pain states. Psychotropic drugs can be defined as agents which affect psychic function, behavior or experience and are most commonly employed in psychiatric practice. In the past few years, however, psychotropic drugs—hypnotics, sedatives, stimulants, antianxiety, and antidepressants—have found a useful place in the treatment of chronic pain.

Table 5–1

SOME DRUGS COMMONLY USED IN TREATING PAIN
(The following medications are registered trademarks.)

Narcotics and Synthetics	*Major Tranquillizers**
Percodan	Haldol
Darvon	Navane
Demerol	Prolixin
Tylenol with Codeine	Thorazine
Talwin	Mellaril

Muscle Relaxants	*Minor Tranquillizers**
Robaxin	Valium
Soma	Librium
Parafon Forte	Tranxene
	Serax

Aspirin Compounds	*Antidepressants*
Excedrin	Sinequan
Alka-Seltzer Pain Reliever	Elavil
Bufferin	Tofranil
Aspirin (Bayer, St. Joseph, etc.)	Norpramine
Ascriptin	Parnate

As discussed in various sections of this text, psychological variables play an important and natural role in our perception of pain. It is not difficult to see how anxiety, tension, depression and frustration gradually become counterparts to the disrupted life-style, disability and suffering of chronic pain. Drugs affecting mood and behavior are frequently used in conjunction with analgesics for the treatment of pain. The contribution of psychotropic agents is the reduction of anxiety, amelioration of depression and improved analgesic effect, often permitting a reduction in dosage of narcotic analgesic drugs. But caution must be taken in the use of psychotropic drugs. In the treatment of chronic pain, prolonged administration of sedative hypnotics and minor tranquillizers alone or in combination with strong analgesics can produce problems with drug dependency. Table 5–2 outlines

---

*The terms major and minor when applied to tranquillizers refer to the chemical structure and action of the tranquillizer and not to the physiological effects that the tranquillizer may produce.

the multiple drug use and abuse of one chronic pain patient. Certain sedatives, for example, may actually reverse the analgesic effect of other medications, so that although the patient may get more sleep, it will be at the expense of feeling greater pain, which in turn may lead to the increased use of analgesic medication. Similarly, prolonged use of a tranquilizer such as Valium® (diazepam) may block the release of serotonin in the brain which interferes with sleep, reduces the body's ability to tolerate pain, and, in some cases, causes depression. Frequently after resolution or remission of a primary pain problem, a residue of drug dependency may complicate matters and supersede pain as the primary medical problem. Although narcotic or sedative addiction *per se* does not generally represent a life-threatening situation, chronic-pain patients may suffer increased depression and anxiety and even increased pain; they may be totally disabled and unable to benefit from programs designed to better manage pain as the result of prolonged use of a variety and quantity of medications.

Table 5–2

MULTIPLE DRUG USE BY MALE SUFFERING BACK PAIN
(The following medications are registered trademarks.)

Drug	*Average Dosage*
1. Librium	10 mg bid PRN
2. Elavil	100 mg hs
3. Darvon N	q6h
4. Serax	25 mg tid PRN
5. Prolixin	2 mg q AM
6. Sinequan	50 mg bid
7. Demerol	50 mg tid PRN
8. Talwin	40 mg q6h PRN
9. Aspirin	6–12 per day

Abbreviations: mg = milligrams
bid = twice a day
tid = three times a day
hs = at bedtime
PRN = as needed
q6h = every 6 hours
qAM = every morning

Valuable and convenient as they are, narcotic and psychotropic drugs do not cure pain, nor can they modify the psychological variables that often contribute to pain. Nonnarcotic drugs such as aspirin are generally thought safe when taken as recommended. In addition, there has been some recent research advocating the efficacy of combining the tricyclic antidepressant Elavil® (amitriptyline) with the phenothiazine major tranquillizer Prolixin® (fluphenazine) in the treatment of chronic pain. Generally speaking, however, the singular or combined use of narcotic and/or psychotropic drugs may effectively reduce the intensity of discomfort in some pain states, but it may also result in mental confusion and even the development of tolerance and dependence. By and large, drugs are far more effective and appropriate for use in acute, temporary pain states than for chronic pain.

CHAPTER SIX

Physical Treatment of Chronic Pain

Many people mistakenly believe that long-term intractable pain is by definition a surgical problem. Indeed, most patients treated at "pain clinics" or "chronic-pain rehabilitation centers" have undergone one or more major surgeries for pain relief. However, there are a number of nonsurgical, nonpharmacological techniques that are often effective in the treatment of chronic pain. Compared to surgery and many types of drugs, the physical techniques to be described in this chapter have several important advantages. The most important such advantage is that physical treatment techniques have a very low risk factor and are nonaddictive.

In this chapter we will discuss several popular physical treatment techniques for pain relief which may be employed prior to surgery as a treatment or diagnostic modality, or following surgery to better rehabilitate the chronic-pain patient and prepare him to return to a more normal life-style.

Transcutaneous Electrical Nerve Stimulation

Electricity's painkilling abilities were well known long before man had any idea what electricity itself was all about, probably as far back as the early Egyptians and the time of Hippocrates. Its first recorded use in that capacity was in 46 A.D. when Scribonius Largus, a Roman physician, used the electric ray or "torpedo fish" for the treatment of headache and gout. Evidently this treatment involved bringing the affected body part in contact with the fish. The electrical jolt would stun the area and relieve the pain, often for hours.

Since this early application, medicine has searched for an effective and practical use of electricity as an anesthetic. The closest we have come to realizing this goal may be transcutaneous electrical nerve stimulation (more commonly referred to as TENS). A TENS unit is basically a battery-powered pulse generator about the size of a pack of cigarettes. A pair of electrodes running from the power unit is attached to the skin directly over the painful area of the body and provides continuous mild electrical stimulation. A low voltage current running between the two electrodes supposedly blocks incoming pain signals travelling along the spinal cord. The technique is reportedly effective in reducing the pain intensity in approximately 35 to 40 percent of those patients treated. Recently, a significant amount of research suggests that TENS may be more effective in acute pain, such as postoperative discomfort than in chronic-pain states, though many pain treatment centers continue to rely heavily on TENS.

Acupuncture

Acupuncture is a highly controversial treatment technique that has gained only limited acceptance in the United States. While this technique has long been an accepted procedure in many Eastern cultures, many non-Easterners consider inserting a needle into one part of the body to relieve pain in another to be quackery and magic. Many Western scientists attribute the value of acupuncture to hypnotic-like suggestion.

Recently, however, a number of Western scientists has postulated a theory to explain the reported effectiveness of acupuncture. They believe that acupuncture alleviates pain not by having a direct effect on the discomfort, but rather by stimulating the nervous system to manufacture its own intrinsic pain-relieving substances, known as endorphins. Other advocates of acupuncture believe that it stimulates certain nerve pathways to send messages to the brain to counteract pain messages. Although there are some doctors and treatment centers that advocate the use of acupuncture, the technique remains highly speculative and experimental.

Nerve Blocks

If your doctor believes that all or part of your pain has resulted from an injured or damaged nerve, he may recommend blocking the nerve in order to interrupt the message of pain carried by the nerve to the brain. "Nerve blocks" are various techniques that involve placing a small-calibre needle through the skin and advancing it to the area of the nerve suspected of contributing to or causing pain. A local anesthetic or alcohol mixture is injected through the needle for the purpose of diagnosis and/or temporary pain relief.

Unfortunately, nerve blocks are not always effective. When they do "take," the relief is only temporary (four to eight hours). Some doctors believe that repeated blocks over a period of weeks can result in prolonged relief from pain, but others question the long-term effectiveness of blocks. Nevertheless, nerve blocks are relatively easy and harmless techniques which have been used for years in selected surgical and obstetrical cases. Besides the pin prick produced by the needle as it punctures the skin, you may expect an occasional muscle twitch or "electricity" feeling in the area of the body affected by the block.

Possible consequences of nerve blocks which you may experience soon after the procedure are dizziness, some shaking and sweating, occasional minor headache, and soreness in the area of the body where the needle has been introduced. Such consequences of nerve-blocking are often caused by various degrees of anxiety and have a tendency to fade out as the nerve-block therapy proceeds.

Other possible consequences of nerve blocks include feelings of warmness, numbness and weakness in the limbs, depending on the bodily region which has been "blocked." If the nerve block involves the face and neck, you may also experience eyelid drop and hoarseness. All of the above feelings are transitory, and recovery can be expected within ten to twelve hours following the procedure.

Other possible, but improbable, complications include various disturbances in vital organ functions and biorhythms, such as changes in breathing, blood pressure and states of awareness. Such complications generally immediately follow the injection of the analgesic drug. Serious side effects of nerve blocks very rarely occur.

Physical Exercise

Physical exercise occupies a special and important place in the treatment of many chronic-pain states. Following an acute injury, most of us protect the affected body part in an effort to reduce pain until the injured area has had time to heal. For example, if you have ever suffered an ankle sprain, you know that putting weight on the injured foot can cause considerable pain. Limping is the body's natural protection device to keep us from further injury and pain until the ankle is healed. If the injury is to the low back, we may move guardedly and slowly, rotating the entire body rather than spontaneously turning and twisting. In addition, because of the pivotal location and function of the lower back, almost all movement results in pain, so we sharply curtail our physical activities. Over time, muscles that are no longer being used and exercised will contract and become weak. Physical conditioning deteriorates and the body becomes "tight." After months of decreased use, muscles become so contracted and weak that their use results in immediate discomfort. By this time the original cause of pain may have healed, yet severe pain on movement is still experienced. However, the etiology of the pain is now weak and contracted muscles and tendons rather than the original injury. Because pain on movement is experienced, we further restrict our motion, and the cycle progresses from bad to worse.

For chronic-pain patients, a graduated program of physical exercise usually results in significant improvement in physiological tone, body strength and functional capacity. Muscles are "stretched" and strengthened in an appropriate program of physical reconditioning designed to work the "kinks" out of the body and restore full range of motion. In addition, exercise is a behavior that is incompatible with pain behavior. As compared to limping, groaning, staying in bed, sitting and guarded movements which can be thought of as "pain behavior," physical exercise is an example of "well behavior." Chapter Nine outlines some physical exercises to help you better manage your pain. Before beginning this or any exercise program following an injury, your doctor should approve your plan for reconditioning.

Occupational Therapy

Occupational therapy can provide a number of valuable services for the chronic-pain patient. Some of these services include evaluating and assessing individual patient needs, such as upper-extremity range of motion and muscle strength; gross and fine coordination skills; sensory, motor and perceptual problems; appropriateness of slings, splints or adaptive equipment; activities of daily living abilities, such as self-care, dressing, bathing and homemaking; and home evaluation with recommendations for adaptive equipment or structural changes. The unique contribution of occupational therapy is that a program of normal activity is used either as a specific treatment or as a simulated work situation to aid in the rehabilitation of the patient. It thus relates to the patient's everyday life and provides the link between medical care and the patient's return to vocational and recreational activity following weeks, months or years of disability.

It is well known that individuals enmeshed in activity temporarily forget their complaints and problems. It is also recognized that physical or mental occupation helps in tolerating pain. This is where occupational therapy fits in and is of particular value to the chronic-pain patient. Occupational therapy involves the patient in enjoyable activities requiring concentration. For example, a dock worker with chronic back pain may be taught ways to bend and lift that create less stress on the spine. His endurance for standing and sitting may be increased by having him work on leather crafts he enjoys. Through gradual exposure, the occupational therapist teaches the patient to emphasize and develop his capabilities and return to a productive life.

Recreational Therapy

The typical chronic-pain patient has suffered months or even years of daily discomfort, frustration and despair, and it is no wonder that most pain victims have long given up recreational interests. Rather than enjoying hobbies and activities, the typical chronic-pain patient searches for relief that seldom comes. As part of the rehabilitation team, recreational therapy attempts to reverse this behavior pattern. Recreational therapy involves gradually exercising and reconditioning patients whose muscles have become weak and stiff from inactivity. In addition, recreational therapy helps the pain victim get his mind off pain and disability by exposing him to a variety of recreational pursuits. Recreational therapy may be the least understood component in the total pain rehabilitation effort, but it serves a highly valuable and professional function.

Physical Therapy

Physical therapy is an important treatment for almost all chronic-pain patients. A physical therapist is a skilled technician who expertly carries out your doctor's orders to exercise and limber tight and painful parts of your body. With chronic-pain patients, physical therapy often involves both treatment and educational components. For example, physical therapy conducts postural instruction and exercises, active exercises (e.g., stretching, postural, bicycle), instruction in body mechanics, flexibility and mobility exercises, teaches relaxation and breathing, and gives instruction in basic anatomy and physiology (which is important in understanding your pain). In addition, physical therapy works closely with your doctor to determine if specific treatment techniques are indicated, such as biofeedback, TENS, cryotherapy (icing), hydrotherapy, ultrasound, massage and hot packs.

Physical medicine techniques play an integral role in the treatment of chronic benign pain, particularly in interdisciplinary pain rehabilitation centers. Chronic pain is not always a surgical problem, and reaching for a pill does not always spell relief. In fact, some doctors and researchers now believe that only a very small select percentage of chronic-pain patients can expect relief from surgical efforts, and prolonged drug use can result in the development of tolerance and dependence. As a result, physical treatment techniques are fast gaining popularity as an alternative and adjunct to surgical and pharmacological treatment of chronic-pain states.

CHAPTER SEVEN

Biofeedback

The term biofeedback has come into popular usage in recent years in both scientific and popular circles. While still in its infancy, a considerable body of scientific research is fast developing which serves to clarify the role of biofeedback in the treatment of chronic pain. First, biofeedback is not a product of our contemporary scientific age but is as old as mankind. Second, biofeedback is not a miracle cure, and it will not revolutionize health care. It will not cure cancer, leukemia, heart disease or the common cold! Biofeedback is simply a treatment technique—a proven, effective treatment technique in carefully selected patients suffering a limited number of medical disorders which have not consistently responded well to traditional medical practices. It is not a "cure-all," but is just one technique in a practitioner's armamentarium.

To understand biofeedback, a careful distinction must first be made between the terms "biofeedback" and "biofeedback training." Biofeedback is a natural, usually unconscious learning process. For example, how did you learn the complex mind—body coordination required to pick up a pencil, to write your name, to walk, to feed yourself without making a mess, to throw a baseball, to play golf or to drive a car? The answer is biofeedback. Through trial-and-error efforts we receive feedback from the environment and our body which we then use to modify and perfect future efforts. For instance, the proper swing of a golf club requires the complex coordination of our muscles, nervous system and sensory systems of sight and touch. Through repeated trial-and-error feedback we refine and improve our coordination and are eventually rewarded with a lower golf score. Slightly more sophisticated types of biofeedback include listening to your heart rate with a stethoscope, weighing yourself on a bathroom scale, taking your blood pressure and taking your temperature with a thermometer. Biofeedback, then, is the measuring or recording of a biological process which is fed back (or made available) to the individual.

If an individual takes a biological process which is measured in some way and continuously "fed back" to him, and he attempts to use the information to guide his trial-and-error efforts to modify a targeted biological process, he is using biofeedback training. For instance, suppose you wanted to learn to decrease your heart rate. You might sit in a chair with a stethoscope to your chest and, through trial and error, attempt different mental strategies until you audibly detected a noticeable decrease. While this is a crude and simplistic example of biofeedback training, it does qualify under our definition. However, if your doctor refers you to a biofeedback specialist for training, don't expect your treatment to be this elementary.

Today biofeedback training for selected medical disorders refers to a variety of techniques utilizing sensitive and highly sophisticated biological recording instruments. To look at a fully equipped biofeedback facility is to be reminded of endless stereo components stacked one on the other with meters, dials and flashing lights. These instruments assist individuals in gaining conscious control over biological processes generally thought not to be under voluntary control. Through electronic measurement, integration, amplification and transformation into easily perceived visual and audio signals, one can sit passively and watch one's blood pressure vary from moment to moment or observe the electrical activity of painful muscles in the neck and back. Combined with other proven effective treatment techniques, biofeedback training is a useful component in the treatment of chronic pain.

Historical Perspective

Scientists and laymen alike have long been fascinated with Far East Yogis who reportedly can walk on broken glass and survive extended periods of time submerged under water without oxygen. The ability to achieve such voluntary control of physiological mechanisms has remained a mystery until about twenty years ago when science began its first serious look at meditation and associated forms of mind–body interactions. Experimentation first began with laboratory animals, but as research and understanding grew, the use of human subjects became commonplace. Let's look at some of the historical highlights in the development of biofeedback from an early mystic phenomenon to an accepted and effective treatment technique.

The roots of the scientific study of biofeedback training can be traced back to the 1960's when Dr. Neil Miller, a psychologist, and his colleagues reported they had successfully trained a number of laboratory rats to voluntarily control their heart rates, blood pressures and formation of urine. Dr. Miller, in fact, claimed that the rats could even be trained to increase the blood flow to one ear while maintaining the natural flow of blood to the other! Needless to say, this report sparked the interest of the scientific community, and the scientifically controlled experimentation of biofeedback began.

Early reports of laboratory animals taught to raise and lower blood pressure, alter blood flow, and increase and decrease their heart rates also met with much skepticism. Biofeedback was in direct contradiction to what had long been accepted as scientific fact: that our bodily processes are controlled by either the voluntary nervous system (e.g., arm and leg movements) or the involuntary nervous system (e.g., heart rate, digestion, blood pressure, etc.). It is true that our hearts will beat without our conscious efforts and that our blood pressure will vary from moment to moment "automatically." However, early biofeedback research demonstrated that we can learn to exert some conscious control over biological processes previously assumed to be totally beyond our control. This was considered a major scientific breakthrough, and the number of researchers investigating biofeedback grew rapidly.

Some twenty years after the beginning of serious scientific investigation of biofeedback, we find that the treatment modality is no longer only speculative laboratory research, but a proven clinical treatment technique. Once a counterculture fad with interest targeted toward achieving nirvana and inner peace through alpha wave feedback, biofeedback training is today performed by thousands of doctors and therapists in treating a variety of chronic-pain conditions such as migraine headaches, tension headaches, low-back pain, Raynaud's disease and temporomandibular joint pain. Biofeedback training has come of age and has gained wide acceptance. But as part of legitimate health care, research efforts must continue to refine the technique and better define the most effective scope of application.

Biofeedback Training: Technique

The most effective use of biofeedback training in the treatment of chronic-pain conditions has focussed on learning voluntary control of one of the following physiological processes: electromyographic biofeedback and thermal biofeedback. Electromyographic (more commonly referred to as EMG) biofeedback is most frequently employed in the treatment of musculoskeletal disorders. Electrical activity of targeted muscle groups is recorded and made continuously available to patients who use this information, along with instructions from the therapist, to gradually learn better control of "tight" or "tense" muscles.

A second frequently employed type of biofeedback in the treatment of chronic pain is known as thermal or temperature biofeedback. Thermal biofeedback is most often the treatment of choice with vascular disorders involving impaired blood circulation in the body, usually the head, hands or feet. Blood flow from an affected body part is recorded and made continuously available to patients who combine the knowledge with instructions from the therapist to increase or decrease circulation to the painful area.

Most patients who undergo biofeedback training are referred by their physician to a biofeedback therapist or doctor who uses biofeedback as one of several techniques in the treatment of chronic pain.* If you are referred for biofeedback

*Unfortunately, neither the Federal Drug Administration nor state governments have yet passed legislation restricting the purchase of biofeedback instruments and the practice of biofeedback training to physicians, clinical psychologists and dentists. As a result, biofeedback techniques are being used by educators, counselors and a host of weakly certified or noncertified medical and psychological therapists. Before treatment, ensure that the practitioner holds a doctorate in medicine, clinical psychology or dentistry.

training, you should remember that biofeedback treatment is much different than other forms of health care to which you may be accustomed. In biofeedback training, the patient must assume responsibility for his health care and expend the effort required to learn and effectively utilize biofeedback skills. Of course, the doctor or therapist will assist you in your training, but the final responsibility falls on the patient. The doctor or therapist acts much like a coach, teaching and directing you as you learn a new skill to combat chronic pain. This approach is in sharp contrast to traditional health care where the doctor assumes responsibility for our health care. Rather than handing you pills to take for your pain, the biofeedback therapist will help you learn ways to manage your pain.

Should you decide that biofeedback is worth a trial, you will learn that biofeedback training involves several phases. The order of the phases and the specifics of treatment will vary with the doctor or therapist and the type of pain you have. However, the following protocol should give you some idea of what to expect from biofeedback training.

The first phase of biofeedback training is termed the baseline phase. After your doctor or biofeedback therapist conducts a careful evaluation of your pain and before feedback training begins, you may be asked to keep a "pain diary" for a week or two. Careful daily charting of your pain intensity and the name and amount of any medication taken will give your doctor or therapist valuable information. For example, in addition to obtaining a baseline measure of your pain intensity and medication intake (which can be used for comparison as you progress in biofeedback training), important pain patterns or trends can often be identified. Baseline measurement prior to beginning biofeedback training is an attempt to provide a degree of control and objectivity to your self-reported pain complaints. It is to the patient's benefit to cooperate and carefully complete the Daily Pain Diary as requested.

Once a baseline has been established, your doctor or therapist will orient you to the biofeedback equipment. You will likely be requested to sit in a comfortable chair, usually located in a dimly lit, sound-resistant room. Your doctor or therapist will explain the operation of the biofeedback equipment, which looks like a collection of stereo components complete with meters, lights and calibration gauges. Depending on where you are experiencing your pain, the skin around the affected body part will be cleaned with alcohol or acetone. This will cleanse the skin of oil and promote the best contact between your skin and the electrodes.

The electrodes (which measure muscle activity or blood flow, depending on the type of biofeedback employed) are next secured to the skin with an adhesive collar. The placement of the electrodes is often directly on the painful body part. Two or three electrodes may be used, with one electrode serving as a ground. You will then be asked to relax while the biofeedback equipment is calibrated and checked.

The next step involves measuring the normal or resting level of the biological process targeted for training. For instance, if your pain problem is chronic muscle-tension headaches, you would be asked to simply relax while the measurement is taken of the muscles in the forehead. This measurement of the resting level is considered a starting point for training. You will gradually learn to control the forehead muscles so that the resting level after successful completion of eight to ten training sessions is greatly decreased when compared to initial pretraining resting levels.

Once a baseline has been established, it is time to begin biofeedback training. The basis of biofeedback is a process known as shaping. Shaping is a basic learning technique whereby progress towards an identified goal is accomplished through small, incremental steps. One step must be successfully mastered before proceeding to the next. Again using muscle-tension headaches as an example, reduced muscle activity or "tightness" is the ultimate goal of EMG biofeedback training. Therefore, your doctor or therapist sets a threshold for you so that a soft tone continuously sounds. Successful muscular relaxation will terminate the tone, thereby signalling that you have successfully decreased your muscle tension. A new threshold for you to work towards is set, and your job is to again terminate the tone by further relaxing your frontalis muscles. Step-by-step levels of muscle tension are decreased through shaping until the patient achieves a resting level of muscle tension which does not result in head pain.

After you begin to demonstrate moderate control of the

targeted biological process, your doctor or therapist may introduce a voluntary control phase to the training protocol. During the voluntary control phase, you will *not* be given feedback. Rather, your doctor or therapist monitors your progress while you exert passive voluntary control of the targeted physiological process. Voluntary control phases instituted in the overall training protocol prohibit excessive dependence on continuous feedback to control biological processes and help generalize the patient's ability to control the targeted process outside of the doctor's office where continuous feedback is not available. When you are able to control successfully the targeted biological process during voluntary control phases, your doctor may ask you to begin practicing your control technique at home between training sessions.

After a number of biofeedback training sessions, which will vary depending on what type of pain you have and how quickly you learn, you should find that your ability to control the targeted response has increased while the time and effort required for voluntary control has decreased. The greater control you develop, the greater effect it should have on your pain. While voluntary control of muscle activity may be relatively easy to learn, control of blood flow may take longer to accomplish and is somewhat more difficult for most people.

Exactly how does one go about learning voluntary control of muscles or blood flow? If you asked most successful biofeedback patients how they voluntarily exercise control over biological processes long thought to be involuntary, they would respond with, "I'm not sure!" Some report relaxing deeply while thinking of their body being warmed by a penetrating heat. Others report conjuring up images of peaceful landscapes. The vast majority, however, report no specific sensation or thought. They describe successful biofeedback control as a "knack" or "sense" that is almost unconsciously produced. They describe it as "will" that, during early training, requires deliberate and careful thought and effort but over time becomes a technique requiring very little consciousness.

Biofeedback with Chronic-Pain States

Biofeedback is currently most widely recognized as effective in the treatment of chronic-pain states. A review of the scientific literature evidences the use of biofeedback in the treatment of a variety of painful medical disorders with varying degrees of success. At this time, it appears that biofeedback training has proven most beneficial in the treatment of migraine and muscle-contraction headaches, low-back pain, Raynaud's disease and temporomandibular joint pain. Let's take a closer look at how biofeedback is effectively utilized in the treatment of these troublesome chronic-pain disorders.

Migraine Headaches

Simply defined, migraine or vascular headache is a disorder characterized by excruciating pain usually located on one side of the head and often accompanied by nausea, vomiting, cognitive impairment, depression, and, occasionally, even suicidal thoughts. Migraine attacks are usually preceded by an aura or prodromal stage during which the victim experiences blurred or double vision, or even temporary blindness. At times there are visions of bright flashing lights, strange shapes or dazzling colors.

A migraine attack usually comes in three states: prodromal, the actual attack and the aftermath. An attack may last anywhere from a few hours to several days, and the pain is nothing less than horrible. Twice as many women suffer migraine headaches as men and, although rare, migraines can affect children as well as adults. Many victims of migraine find that the attacks cease to occur when they reach middle age, although other victims endure migraines all their lives.

A fortunate discovery at the Menninger Foundation in Topeka, Kansas, in the late Sixties led to the development of the thermal biofeedback technique of treating migraines. During tests of the ability to learn control of blood flow to the extremities, a subject who happened to be experiencing a migraine at the time of the investigation reported an unexpected side effect. The subject claimed that she experienced a sudden decrease in the intensity and severity of her headache, which the researchers noted coincided with a dramatic increase in the blood flow to the subject's hands. This discovery was the catalyst for an intensive five-year study of thermal biofeedback as a treatment technique for migraine headaches.

Thermal biofeedback involves attaching a small, sensitive

thermometer to the tip of the index finger. The thermometer measures the warmth of the skin, the skin temperature being associated with blood flow. In other words, the greater the warmth of the hands, as measured by a special thermometer, the greater the blood flow to the extremities. The patient is instructed to watch a meter that gives continuous visual feedback of hand temperature. Through trial-and-error prac- tice and with instructions from the doctor or therapist, the patient soon learns to increase the warmth of the hands, thereby increasing the blood flow to the hands. After several training sessions, many patients learn to increase the warmth of their hands by as much as 8–10°F (about 4°C). Of course, voluntary control of extremity blood flow is associated with a decrease in frequency, intensity, and duration of migraine attacks.

Research and clinical results of thermal biofeedback effec- tiveness in the treatment of migraine headaches have been mixed. While some studies report that as many as 60 to 80 percent of patients benefit from thermal biofeedback, perhaps a more accurate estimate may be closer to 40 or 50 percent. However, when thermal biofeedback is combined with relaxa- tion exercises and modifications in life-style, the technique offers hope to many migraine victims who otherwise continue to suffer despite the best efforts of medical science.

Muscle-Contraction Headaches

The advertising world does not hesitate to suggest possible reasons and remedies for muscle-contraction (ten- sion) headaches. We usually are shown a stress situation, such as a housewife rushing to prepare dinner while two or three children scream and cry, the telephone rings, the doorbell rings and the roast beef burns. The frantic housewife clutches her head in obvious distress as the television announcer rec- ommends taking Brand X pills "for fast headache relief." In reality, this often does prove to be the case. Many of us are subject to occasional headaches when there is unusual pres- sure at home or work, when we are enduring a particularly frustrating period, or suffering from glare combined with heat. For this type of occasional head pain, "Brand X" analgesic pills probably work well. But what if the headaches occur more and more frequently, even daily, and the consumption of analgesics creeps up steadily? Medical attention is then usually required.

Tension headaches affect both sides of the head symmetrically in approximately 90 percent of tension-headache patients, unlike migraine which is usually located only on one side of the head. The quality of the headache is remarkably consistent and characteristic. It is often described as a tightness, more of an uncomfortable feeling of pressure than pain. It is also described as a dull ache in the forehead, or the temples, or the back of the head, or the neck, or even "all over the head." Approximately one in ten muscle-contraction-headache sufferers also is plagued with vascular involvement. Known as "combined muscle contraction–migraine" headaches, the disorder appears to be a link between the two maladies and frequently complicates an accurate diagnosis.

The victim of chronic tension headaches experiences pain not only during tense or stressful situations, but also may endure head pain in anticipation of any unpleasantness. The symptoms may later begin in advance of a day's work, a routine shopping trip, a visit to friends or any of the other aspects of daily life. In time, the patient's activity level and optimism decrease as the consumption of analgesic medication increases. The product is a distressing cycle of chronic pain and, as a result, further muscle tension and pain. Tense muscles cause pain because prolonged muscle constriction depletes the muscle of oxygen and decreases blood flow. As a result, toxins build up in muscle tissue, resulting in pain.

Biofeedback treatment of muscle-contraction headaches is based on the following premise: If muscular tension in the shoulders, neck and head can be decreased or prevented before it begins, and can be maintained at reduced levels, headache frequency can be reduced or even eliminated. Muscles give off electrical discharges which can be measured and recorded with biofeedback instruments. Electrodes are attached to the frontalis muscles in the forehead or to the neck and shoulders. The patient then uses continuous audio or visual feedback of muscle activity to learn techniques to reduce muscular tension. Specific relaxation exercises (Chapter

Ten) are frequently included as part of the treatment regimen, and successful elimination of tension headaches can usually be accomplished within five to ten training sessions. Once treatment ends, the patient must continue home practice of the relaxation technique to guard against relapse.

Low-Back Pain

Biofeedback training for chronic low-back pain is one of the newest and least documented uses of biofeedback training. Nevertheless, research is continuing, and early controlled outcome studies appear promising. Most recent investigations suggest that the effectiveness of biofeedback training for back pain is greatly facilitated when feedback is combined with other treatment techniques, such as physical therapy, medication, psychotherapy, physical exercises and relaxation exercises. Although debate continues, many clinicians believe that the value of EMG biofeedback in the treatment of low-back pain is general muscular relaxation. Electrodes are secured to the area of the lumbar spine and feedback of muscle activity is given to the patient who practices techniques to lower muscular tension.

Raynaud's Disease

Raynaud's disease is a relatively rare disorder caused by an abnormal degree of spasm of the blood vessels in the extremities, leading to pale, cold and extremely painful fingers or toes. It is generally believed to be triggered by cold temperatures and/or stress. Because of vascular spasms, blood flow to the affected body part is greatly reduced, causing the fingers or toes to become blanched and cold to the point where even the motion required to pick up a pencil can cause excruciating extremity pain. Traditional medical treatment for this disorder includes vasodilating drugs and keeping the hands and feet as warm as possible.

You may suspect from our previous discussion of biofeedback training for migraine headaches that thermal or temperature biofeedback might be an effective treatment for Raynaud's disease as well. Remember that thermal biofeedback involves learning to "warm the hands" by increasing the blood flow to the extremities. Research documents that thermal biofeedback is indeed an effective and useful technique for managing the pain of Raynaud's disease. As in the case of migraine treatment, a specially designed supersensitive thermometer is attached to the index finger (or the big toe, depending on which extremity is causing pain). Blood flow is then measured and fed back to the patient who, through trial-and-error, gradually learns techniques to increase blood flow. Eight to twelve training sessions are usually required to learn to increase the blood flow to cold, painful and circulatory impaired fingers and toes.

Temporomandibular Joint Pain

Temporomandibular joint (TMJ) pain is a stress-related muscular spasm of the cheek and jaw area just in front of the ear. Occasionally the pain radiates from the jaw through the neck to the shoulders or even to the mid-back. Victims of TMJ pain describe the discomfort as a steady, dull, intense pain that can last for hours without relief. Because the pain radiates from the masseter muscle of the jaw, dentists normally first diagnose and treat the disorder by using a variety of techniques including mouth guards, surgery and local anesthetics. Unfortunately, since the pain is caused by muscular tension resulting from clenching the jaw during stressful periods, mouth guards and surgery do little to decrease the pain, and anesthetics provide only temporary relief.

EMG biofeedback training in the treatment of TMJ pain has proven very successful, especially when feedback training is combined with relaxation exercises. Electrodes are attached to the affected muscle site and feedback is given to the patient. The patient gradually learns, through practice and shaping, to decrease muscular tension and, consequently, relieve the pain. Generally, six to ten training sessions are required to master this technique.

CHAPTER EIGHT

Hypnosis

For the vast majority of people today, "hypnosis" still is thought of as a weird, if not demonic and frightening, occult art. Individuals who practice hypnosis are frequently thought to exert mystical dominance over their subjects, who are rendered powerless to resist. Others may be considered charlatans, whose sole function is to provide entertainment to crowds who laugh uproariously as subjects skip across a stage barking like dogs or scream in terror at invisible snakes.

Yet, despite deep-rooted prejudices, hypnosis has gradually gained more acceptance in recent years as a valid and useful medical and psychological treatment technique. There now exists a significant body of research that documents the effectiveness of hypnosis in the treatment of pain in such disorders as burns, anxiety, cancer, tension, arthritis, leukemia, menstrual discomfort, ulcers, postoperative pain and nausea, childbirth, neck and lower-back pain, headaches, dental procedures and more!

Why, then, has acceptance of hypnosis come so slowly, both from the public and scientific communities? Undoubtedly the answer is complex, but two important factors deserve discussion. First, it is not understood how hypnosis works. It should quickly be added, however, that it is not known how many of the major analgesic medications work, either. The practice of medicine is not an exact science. For example, not only are we unable to cure cancer, leukemia and many other serious illnesses, but we also do not have the knowledge of disease and pharmacology necessary to cure the common cold! Just as it isn't necessary to understand fully the mechanics of an automobile engine to drive a car, neither is it necessary to understand fully why and how hypnosis works in order to reap the benefits of this proven effective treatment technique. Perhaps it is wise to remember Hippocrates' statement about the art of medicine, that "nothing should be omitted in an art which interests the whole world, especially something that may be beneficial to suffering humanity and which does not risk human life or comfort."

A second factor that has hindered the acceptance of hypnosis as legitimate treatment has been the many misconceptions harbored by both the public and professional communities. Maybe the most common of these is that when a person is hypnotized, he is actually unconscious. This idea frightens many people, since one of our deepest and most dreaded fears is that of losing control and looking foolish. In reality, nothing could be farther from the truth. Even in the deeper stages of hypnosis, the patient remains alert. He can hear the doctor's voice and can verbally communicate. He can answer questions, respond in a rational and lucid manner, and be fully aware of what is going on. In fact, if the doctor does not carefully explain the subtle signs that indicate when a patient is hypnotized, the subject may deny that he was ever "in a trance," since he was fully aware of everything that was said and done. Only in the very deepest stage of hypnosis is the patient amnesic on awakening.

Another widespread misconception is that only a very select few individuals can be hypnotized. While everyone is not susceptible to the deepest stages of hypnosis, almost everyone can be hypnotized to some depth of trance. A number of clinicians believe the following figures represent a general consensus of susceptibility to hypnosis: unable to be hypnotized, 5 percent; light trance, 40 percent; medium trance, 45 percent; deep trance, 10 percent.

Yet another misconception is the belief that if a person can be hypnotized, it indicates a personal weakness or personality flaw. Hypnotic induction depends to a great extent on the ability of the patient to concentrate and utilize vivid and graphic mental imagery—characteristics generally believed to be correlated with a high level of intelligence. Hypnosis can only be achieved with the intelligent cooperation of the patient; for that reason, emotionally stable and intelligent persons make the best subjects. In fact, many clinicians believe that hypnosis should not be attempted with persons suffering from select personality disorders, neurosis or a suspected or diagnosed psychosis.

A fourth misconception about hypnosis is that a person is never quite the same after he has been hypnotized. Some people even believe that hypnosis causes a change in brain cell composition and thereby results in organic damage. This, of course, is not true. While there is no full explanation of why and how hynosis works, there is absolutely no evidence to suggest that it causes any structural or organic damage.

Another misconception some people have is that the hypnotist can fully control the subject while the subject is under hypnosis. It is not uncommon to hear the layman hypothesize that a group of criminals could hypnotize an innocent victim and force him, under hypnosis, to rob a bank or maybe even kill someone. It is also not uncommon to see magazine advertisements urging the reader to send money for a home-study course in how to hypnotize subjects without their knowledge or cooperation, sensationalism being a major part of these advertisements. The simple fact is, subjects will not engage in any behavior under hypnosis that they would refuse to do otherwise. We have already noted that even in the deeper stages of hypnosis, the subject remains alert and conscious. If a hypnotized person is given an objectionable suggestion, he will either refuse to engage in the behavior or will voluntarily bring himself out of the hypnotic trance. No control is associated with hypnosis—only suggestion.

The History of Hypnosis

So far as we can tell from recorded history, hypnosis has always played some part in human life, though the term itself has only been in existence for slightly over one hundred years. Witch doctors, medicine men and priests were among the early practitioners. In China, Wang Tai, the "father of Chinese medicine" (whose teachings are still used today), wrote in 2600 B.C. about medical treatment using incantations and mysterious passes over the patient, leaving no doubt about the hypnotic value of these actions. In 1500 B.C., the Veda (the sacred literature of the Hindus) mentioned the use of hypnosis, and the Ebers Papyrus, which is over three thousand years old, described a hypnotic technique very similar to one that is popular today. In the Bible, both in the Old and New Testaments, there are many references to the use of suggestion and hypnosis by mortal man in the treatment of diseases that today might be classified as conversion hysteria or psychosomatic disorders.

The story of modern medical hypnosis can be said to have begun over two hundred years ago in eastern Switzerland. A Roman Catholic priest named Father Gassner effectively used hypnosis in the treatment of hundreds of men and women "possessed of the devil," according to the general belief of that time.

In 1775, Franz Anton Mesmer, a German physician who had heard of Father Gassner's healing powers, arrived in Switzerland. After numerous demonstrations, Mesmer formulated a theory to explain this powerful phenomenon: The body must have two poles, and it transfers some invisible magnetic fluid between the poles. In other words, the body operates like a magnet. Disease was presumably the result of an interruption in the flow of magnetic fluid and could be cured by correcting the invisible flow.

Mesmer believed that only a select few were gifted to be able to control the transmission of magnetic fluid, and for the technique to be effective there must exist a close interest and sympathy between the hypnotist and the patient. He termed the relationship between the healer and the patient *rapport*, a French word meaning harmony or connection. This term continues to be popular today among psychologists and psychiatrists when describing a therapeutic relationship between doctor and patient.

As Mesmer's fame grew, he soon found himself unpopular among his colleagues who had no understanding or interest in hypnosis. His colleagues were at last successful in persuading the Viennese Medical Council to brand him a fraud. Mesmer then left Vienna for Paris where he continued to practice what he termed "animal magnetism" until his death.

News of hypnosis soon spread to England. In the 1830's, a physician named John Elliotson began experimenting on patients he thought might benefit from such treatment. Dr. Elliotson was most successful, and his dramatic cures elicited great interest among both students and colleagues. Unfortunately, the fate of Dr. Elliotson was not unlike that of Mesmer's in Vienna more than a century before. His colleagues forced him to resign his hospital appointment and terminate his practice of medicine. We recognize today that Dr. Elliotson was the first doctor we know of that formulated a list of specific symptoms and disorders which responded particularly well to hypnosis.

While Dr. Elliotson was developing his own theories, a doctor named James Esdaile founded, with the financial assistance of the British government, the first hospital devoted to hypnotic healing in Calcutta, India, in the 1830's. Dr. Esdaile immediately began an investigation of hypnotic anesthesia (certainly there was a great need since chloroform and ether had not yet been discovered). He conducted thousands of operations using hypnotic anesthesia: over three hundred major surgeries including nineteen limb amputations. According to historians, these surgeries were all performed without any sensation of pain. Dr. Esdaile is credited with being the first to recognize the relationship that exists between hypnosis and the perception of pain—a relationship that today forms the basis of our use of hypnosis in the treatment of chronic pain.*

What Is Hypnosis?

Remember the fable of the four blind men asked to describe an elephant? Each man touched a different part of the elephant's anatomy and described the animal accordingly. Much like the elephant, hypnosis has been described in so many ways that one wonders if there are as many definitions as there are definers. Of the countless theories proposed to explain hypnosis, the majority fall into one of the three following groupings: Pavlovian theory, psychoanalytic theory and experimental theory.

Pavlovian Theory

Ivan Pavlov, a Russian scientist best known for his utilization of salivating dogs to demonstrate how some forms of learning take place, believed that hypnosis was a state between wakefulness and sleep. This school theorizes that lower brain-stem

* Hypnotic control of pain is one of the oldest and most enduring uses of hypnosis, yet the reader should be warned. Control of pain with hypnosis should be done only by clinical psychologists, dentists and physicians who are aware of the complex diagnostic and treatment problems of organic illnesses.

portions of the brain were involved in a subject entering a hypnotized state. In other words, during hypnosis a part of the brain becomes inhibited in such a way as to resemble normal sleep, while other portions of the cortex remain alert and enable the hypnotist to maintain contact with the patient.

Pavlovian theory remains alive and well, and there are some modern researchers who continue to subscribe to it. However, most recognized authorities do not believe that there is any similarity between sleep and hypnosis. These researchers point to the evidence that during normal sleep, suggestibility is markedly decreased, rapport is lost and memories are eliminated. A hypnotized person is far more alert to his environment than when he is asleep. In fact, it seems that the whole concept of sleep, when applied to hypnosis, obscures rather than clarifies the issue.

Psychoanalytic Theory

The chief spokesman for this school was Sigmund Freud, who believed that hypnosis represents a separation between the *ego* and the external world. Briefly, the ego is that part of our personality which is in contact with the reality of the external world and which serves to mediate between primitive, instinctual *id* needs and the civilized, moralistic *superego*. It is a hypothetical construct (i.e., a hypothesized structure that does not physically exist). During hypnosis, it is proposed to the patient that he become progressively more oblivious of external stimuli, except those produced by the hypnotist. This is explained by assuming that there exists in the brain a central zone of cortical excitement, surrounded by a zone of cortical inhibition. The patient then turns his thoughts inward until he regresses to an infantile state. The patient responds to hypnotic suggestions because he attributes to the hypnotist the role of parent. In other words, like all children, the patient wants to please his parents (hypnotist), and the hypnotist tells him that his pain is decreased and more under voluntary control. There is even less support among researchers for this theory than for the Pavlovian theory.

Experimental Theory

In contrast to Pavlovian and psychoanalytic theories, which are primarily based on "armchair theorizing," a number of theories about hypnosis have come from experimental laboratories and are supposedly based on controlled scientific investigation. For example, until very recently, one of the major theoretical issues in hypnosis was whether hypnosis led to a unique or altered state of consciousness. T.X. Barber has been a firm believer that hypnosis is not an altered state of consciousness, and supports this opinion with experimental evidence. For instance, under hypnosis it is possible to give a person the suggestion that he is deaf, and the subject will not respond to noise. Barber believed that the hypnotic state was not responsible for the deafness and, in fact, hypothesized that these persons can hear, but they just do not respond to noise. To investigate, Barber used delayed auditory feedback (a procedure whereby a person wearing earphones speaks and hears his voice simultaneously). In delayed auditory feedback, the voice feedback is delayed a fraction of a second so that the person hears what he has just said rather than what he is saying. An individual with normal hearing will quickly become confused and begin to mispronounce words, while a deaf person is not affected. Barber has shown that hypnotized persons behave more like people with normal hearing than like deaf people under delayed auditory feedback: They begin to stammer and their speech slows down. According to Barber, this indicates they hear the stimulus.

If hypnosis is not a trancelike state, then what kind of state is it? Barber believes being under hypnosis is like becoming engrossed in an interesting novel, play or movie. When watching a highly suspenseful movie, for example, we become totally involved in the drama and experience all the emotion contained in the movie. According to Barber, it is just as misleading to explain the experiences of the hypnotized subject by saying that he is in a hypnotic trance as it is to explain the experiences of the movie viewer by saying that he is in a hypnotic trance.

We have briefly looked at the three major theories defining hypnosis and found each to be riddled with controversy. It seems that we are back again to the fable of the four blind men asked to describe an elephant—hypnosis has been described in vastly different ways, depending on what aspect of hypnosis one examines. Like the elephant, hypnosis is just too big and involved a subject to be described accurately by focussing all of our attention to only one specific aspect.

The Hypnotic Experience

The hypnotic experience can be thought of as a continuum, ranging from a very light stage which we can drift into without even being aware of it, to the deepest stages which may appear similar to a sleepwalker's state of consciousness. The lightest stages of hypnosis seem almost like a game that the brain plays on us. Perhaps you can remember times when your gaze seemed drawn to some blank wall or even into space and your mind seemed totally blank. Maybe your breathing became full and slow, your heart rate decreased and your muscles seemed unusually relaxed. You felt calm, tranquil and totally at peace.

When you snapped back to reality you felt as if you had been a million miles from earth, although you remembered exactly what you were thinking and feeling. The feeling is similar to that sensation experienced just before falling asleep, except that rather than feeling dulled and hazy, our concentration seems crystal clear!

The middle or intermediate stage of hypnosis is characterized by the increased intensity of those sensations experienced in the lightest stage. The body feels even more peaceful and relaxed, while the mind seems more alert and clearer than ever. During this stage we also become more susceptible to suggestion. The body and mind seem free from the limitations of everyday living, and we are more fully able to achieve our true physical and mental capabilities. Frequently, we find that an arm or leg can be extended for prolonged periods of time without strain or fatigue. We may even sense that time has stopped, or is speeding rapidly by; that a stationary object is moving, or that a once painful area of the body is now less painful or pain-free.

Individuals susceptible to the intermediate stage of hypnosis will often report being completely aware of what they were doing and feeling unusually calm, relaxed and confident that they could achieve whatever the hypnotist suggested. These individuals frequently report a feeling of confidence that they could bring themselves out of the hypnotic state at will.

The deepest stage of hypnosis is sometimes termed somnambulism and is best described as being similar to a sleepwalker's state of consciousness. This stage is characterized by an even more powerful intensity of those perceptual and physical sensations common in the light and intermediate stages of hypnosis. For example, in the deepest stage of hypnosis, mental acuity may be so concentrated as to enable the person to recall past events that have long been forgotten or suppressed. The technique of age regression, so popular in the media, can occasionally be accomplished in the somnambulistic stage. Needless to say, susceptibility to suggestion is greatly enhanced in the deepest stage, and individuals returning to normal consciousness from somnambulistic hypnosis occasionally report no memory of their thoughts or actions during the session. It is generally agreed that only about one in ten individuals is susceptible to the somnambulistic stage.

It is important to understand that the stages of hypnosis are not as clearly defined as this presentation may appear. While in a light stage of hypnosis, some individuals experience the perceptual and physical sensations common in the deepest stage. Again, it is best that one thinks of hypnosis as a flexible continuum rather than as three separate and distinct stages and realize that the therapeutic effects of hypnosis do not depend on the depth of the hypnotic state. Many individuals are able to control pain while in a light hypnotic stage. In fact, major surgical procedures have been performed on selected individuals who were particularly susceptible to the hypnotically induced absence of the normal sense of pain (hypnoanalgesia) while in a light hypnotic stage.

How Hypnosis Works

As mentioned, no one knows exactly how hypnosis works, but we do know three general components that appear to be most important in successful hypnosis: concentration, suggestibility and imagination. Successful hypnotic induction depends, to a great extent, on the voluntary cooperation of the patient who is asked to concentrate intently on the suggestions of the doctor. The ability to concentrate deeply varies among individuals, but it is most likely to be found in people who readily accept the fact that there are several states of consciousness. How well can you concentrate? Are you able to shut out the distractions of the day when you go to bed at night? Can you read a book in a noisy dormitory or when the television is blaring?

A second important component of hypnosis may be termed suggestibility—meaning that hypnosis tends to be most effective if you expect it to be. Some people feel that suggestibility is a negative trait. Perhaps they equate being suggestible with being naive or gullible. This is unfortunate, for suggestibility is a positive and important trait in hypnosis.

During hypnosis the patient may receive a suggestion from the doctor that he is engaged in some other mental or physical activity that is incompatible with the problem behavior. To illustrate, let's imagine a patient with chronic neck pain that's been described as cold, shooting pains up the back of the neck. During hypnosis, the doctor may suggest that the patient is experiencing a warm, relaxed feeling through the neck and head rather than cold, shooting pain. As the neck and head warm, the pain gradually subsides, and the experience of pain is replaced by an experience of relaxed warmth. Though the patient's central nervous system continues to receive pain impulses, his concentration has been diverted to the feelings of warmth and muscle relaxation. Remember, pain exists only if it is perceived!

A third component of hypnosis is imagination. Do you have a vivid and strong imagination? If you were asked to sit quietly, close your eyes, and imagine floating high above the ground on a giant pillowy white cloud, could you do it? Would you feel that texture of the cloud against your skin? Would you look far below and see the green treetops and the colors of the landscape? Would you close your eyes and feel a warm breeze gently blowing your cloud across the sky? The ability to create rich, vivid mental images may be more closely related to hypnotic susceptibility than any other characteristic.

In summary, research suggests that those who benefit most from hypnosis tend to be able to concentrate well and are suggestible, imaginative and truly motivated to seek relief from their pain. Is this an accurate description of you? If so, then the chances are excellent that you will be a good candidate for hypnotic pain control. If you're in doubt, why not give it a try and see if hypnosis can help you to better modify your pain.

Hypnotic Strategies

Should you decide to pursue hypnosis, ask your doctor to refer you to a competent clinical psychologist or psychiatrist who specializes in the treatment of chronic pain. Here is what you may expect.

First, you will probably be asked to sit in a comfortable chair and relax while the light in the room is slightly lowered to reduce distraction. While we generally think of lying down to relax, research has indicated that hypnosis is best achieved when the patient is sitting up. Next, you will be reminded that pain exists only if it is perceived, and you will be asked to concentrate intently on what the hypnotist says. The particular hypnotic strategy that your doctor employs depends on the preference of the doctor. There is a near-endless number of strategies targeted towards the modification of physical pain.

How long the effects of hypnosis last, as well as the degree of its effectiveness, will vary from individual to individual. Some patients are fortunate enough to receive relief for weeks at a time, while others may require frequent hypnotic suggestion in much the same way that analgesic medication is taken.

An interesting example of the use of hypnosis in the treatment of chronic pain was reported by Dr. Lewis B. Sachs and his colleagues at the Stanford Research Institute.* In this study, eight patients with various types of chronic pain were treated with hypnosis. The results indicated that hypnosis was effective in reducing the intensity of pain, the levels of depression, hypochondriasis and hysteria, and the disruption of sleep, social relations and daily activities. For six of the eight patients, analgesic medication, including Demerol® and codeine, was significantly reduced and three of the patients stopped their medication.

Hypnosis is a proven effective treatment technique for many sufferers of chronic pain, but it is not ideal for everyone. Fortunately, there are a variety of other pain-control treatments available. In fact, most doctors who specialize in the treatment of chronic pain consider hypnosis as but one treatment technique in a multimodal treatment program. Other techniques may include behavior therapy, biofeedback, specialized forms of physical therapy, relaxation training, psychotherapy and the reduction of medication.

American Journal of Clinical Hypnosis, Vol. 20, 1977, p. 106–113.

CHAPTER NINE

Care for the
Aching Back

Few people go through life without experiencing back pain at one time or another. In fact, 80 percent of us will have a severe backache sometime during our lives. Back trouble is one of the most common causes of doctor visits in the United States and the leading cause of long-term disability and absenteeism from work. On any given day, it is estimated that more than seven million men and women are receiving medical treatment for back pain. Over one million workers are absent from their jobs during each year because of back injuries. Backache alone costs employers over one billion dollars annually in sick pay and wages for replacement personnel.*

What is even more staggering than the statistics cited above is this: Ninety percent of all back pain is preventable! Our own deliberate or accidental abuse frequently causes the problem— usually through faulty posture, inactivity, poor physical habits, tension and improper mattresses, chairs and shoes. The number of back injuries is high and is increasing each year. Better prevention and relief from back pain can be achieved if we understand the principles of body mechanics and are aware of our physical limits and capabilities.

PREVENTING BACK PAIN

The best cure for back trouble is to avoid having back trouble. Faulty posture and poor physical conditioning alone account

*"Behavior Modification Can Cure Back Pain," Occupational Health and Safety, Vol. 45, 1976, p. 28–29.

for much of the back pain that Americans experience. To be the one person out of five who avoids acute back pain, consider this simple suggestion: Think about your back during your daily activities.

Posture

Most of us sit in furniture designed for attractiveness rather than proper body support, drive the half-mile to the post office rather than walk, take the elevator up one or two floors, sit behind a desk all day, wear stylish shoes such as loafers and high-heels, and carry a twenty-pound briefcase around several hours each day.

Standing

Slouchers are easy targets for back trouble. When the shoulders are slumped, the pelvis tilts forward, the ribs point downward, the chin is out and the lower spine is swayback. This posture not only crowds and pushes the internal organs together, but it may also strain muscles and ligaments.

Just as slouching or slumped posture is asking for back trouble, so too is the exaggerated military posture many of us were told was the correct way to stand. Military "attention" posture forces the shoulders too far back, and the muscles are held too tightly. The worst part, however, is the curve that such rigid posture creates in the small of the back.

The best way to stand is relaxed, with your head straight, chin slightly tucked, stomach in, and the buttocks tucked under. While the spine is never perfectly straight, this relaxed posture, combined with a slight backward tilt, straightens the spine to its most natural curve and also provides relief from ligament and muscle strain.

When you must stand for long intervals, put one foot on a stool. Every few minutes put the other foot up; alternate. Prolonged standing fatigues the hip muscles and slowly pulls the pelvis forward. This creates an unnatural curve in the lower spine and strains the lower-back muscles. Placing a foot on a stool counteracts this stress by returning the spine to its natural shape.

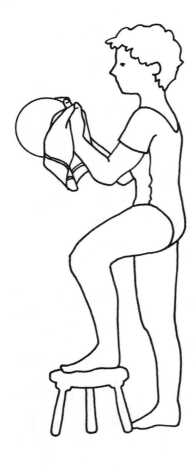

To counteract stress on the lower-back muscles resulting from prolonged standing, place one foot on a stool. Every few minutes, put the other foot up; alternate.

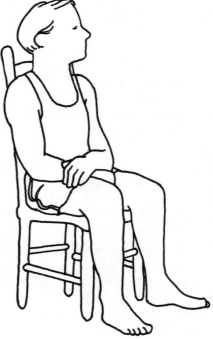

When sitting, your knees should be level with or slightly higher than your hips. Keep your feet flat on the floor.

Sitting

Sitting is more stressful to your back than standing because the spine is no longer balanced on the pelvis. When seated, the pelvis tends to tilt backwards, flattening the normal curve of the lower spine. After a period of time, ligaments and muscles in the back begin to protest. Avoid stuffy chairs that sink in with your weight to mould your body shape. It is also best to avoid chairs that force you to sit in awkward positions (such as beanbag chairs).

If your job requires a great deal of sitting, choose a chair that hugs the small of your back. Adjust the height of the chair so the knees are level with or slightly higher than your hips, and keep both feet flat on the floor. Crossing your legs tilts the pelvis forward much the same way that prolonged standing does and is murder on the back.

Never sit for more than an hour without walking around and stretching. Balancing the books of a multimillion-dollar company or the family checkbook requires intense concentration and creates generalized muscle tension. A quick walk every hour to the office water fountain or the family kitchen will help relax your muscles and your mind.

Driving an automobile can also be hazardous to your back if you do not sit properly. Adjust the seat so your feet can reach the pedals without stretching your legs. Sports cars are built low to the ground and require that your legs be straight, straining the muscles in the lower back. If you drive a lot, buy a firm supportive backrest. It is also a good idea to pull off the road every hour or so to get out of the car and stretch. Your back will thank you!

Sleeping

The key to proper sleeping habits is the knees. Bending the knees unlocks the spine into a neutral position and relieves ligament and muscle stress. Since most of us spend as much as one-third of our lives sleeping, proper sleeping posture is very important in the care of the back.

Start with a firm mattress. As in sitting, the spine should be supported in a neutral position. This requires a firm mattress to prevent sagging. It is not necessary to buy a special orthopedic mattress unless your doctor recommends it. Almost any mattress can be made firm enough by putting a plywood board under it.

There are two proper positions for sleeping. The first is on your back. If you are comfortable sleeping on your back, place a pillow or cushion under your knees to bend the knees. This will neutralize the swayback that is created when you lie flat with your legs straight.

If you are more comfortable on your side, this position is fine, too. Use a pillow under your head so that your neck is properly aligned with your spine. Next, bend the knees to neutralize spinal stress and place a pillow between the knees to keep from twisting the lower back.

Now some "don't's" about proper sleeping posture. First, don't sleep on your stomach. This position causes swayback and increased muscle and ligament stress. Second, don't sleep on a waterbed. Waterbeds do not provide proper firmness and support for the spine. Finally, don't prop yourself up to read in bed. This causes an unnatural curve in the spine and spells disaster for the back.

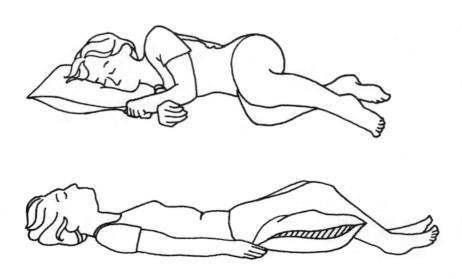

Lifting

Probably more back injuries result from improper lifting than from any other single activity. Since most backaches result from minor injuries, careful lifting will eliminate many problems.

When lifting, let the legs do the work. Weightlifters know the proper posture for lifting is bending the knees and keeping the back straight. Position your body with one foot ahead of the other for balance and pull the object close to your body before lifting it. If you bend from the waist with your legs straight, you may someday find it impossible to get back up again! Grasp the object firmly and lift with the legs, keeping the object close to the body and lifting it no higher than your waist. Never turn from the waist. Instead, turn from the feet or point the forward foot in the direction of the turn in order to reduce twisting of the body. Heavy objects should be set down the same way.

Think again about your back when lifting luggage, tying shoes and raking leaves. Never reach into the backseat or trunk of a car to lift a heavy suitcase. When tying your shoes, squat rather than bend at the waist. Finally, rake leaves from left-to-right or right-to-left; never stretch forward to pull the leaves towards your feet.

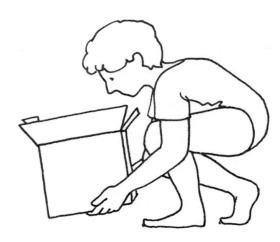

Bending

Bending at the waist should be avoided whenever possible since bending throws the distribution of body weight off balance. Body weight is balanced on the pelvis which acts as a fulcrum for the upper and lower body. Bending tilts this balance and places a strain on the discs, muscles and ligaments that support the spine.

What do you do if you drop the car keys on the floor? *Squat* rather than bend, keeping the back in a vertical position. Squatting uses the leg muscles rather than the back muscles. Since muscles in the lower back may be no bigger than your finger and muscles in the legs may be as big as your wrist, squatting can prevent a painful back injury.

When you buy a new vacuum cleaner, take it for a practice spin and check to see if you can use it without stooping. If you're already saddled with the wrong kind, bend your knees slightly while vacuuming rather than stooping over. If you decide to do some minor mechanical repairs on your car, lie across the fender rather than bending over it, especially if you aren't accustomed to regularly bending over an automobile engine. While making beds, do a few knee bends to tuck in the corners and walk around the bed. Don't reach for the opposite corner of a queen-sized bed. Finally, adjust the lawn-mower handles to your height, so you are not bending over to grasp them.

EXERCISE

Strong and properly conditioned muscles are essential to proper back care. They support the spinal column and determine posture, which is essential for a healthy back. If the muscles are weak, not only are you more likely to suffer a back injury, but recovery will be more difficult.

Regular participation in sports and other forms of active exercise will strengthen your back and condition the rest of your body as well. Everyone can exercise, although your doctor should be consulted if you are in poor physical condition. Back exercises need not involve organized sports and can be done alone in your office or home. Before attempting any exercise program, remember the following:

1. Do not get carried away in an enthusiastic exercise effort. Be realistic and keep in mind your physical condition. Start at a

low degree of difficulty and exertion and gradually progress to more strenuous and lengthy exercises.

2. Work out slowly and easily, and do not try to push over your limit. Exercise only until your muscles become comfortably tired. Your endurance will build in time.

3. Get into an exercise habit. Exercising a little every day is better than doing a lot at one time. Pick times to do your back exercises on a daily schedule.

Pelvic Roll

The pelvic roll is a rotation exercise for the joints in the spine and is an excellent exercise for backache. Lie on your back with your arms straight out to the sides. Bend the knees and place the feet on the floor as near your buttocks as is comfortable. Keeping your arms out to your sides for balance, rock your knees side to side in an easy and smooth rhythm.

Bend-Sitting

Bend-sitting exercises stretch and relax muscles and ligaments in the lower back. Sit on a straight chair with your hands folded in your lap. Bend forward, bringing the chin between your knees. Hold for a count of ten, return to the starting position while tensing the abdominal muscles, relax a moment, and then repeat.

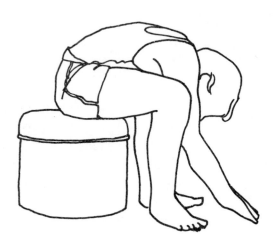

Pelvic Tilt

The pelvic tilt exercise strengthens the muscles in the lower back that control the pelvis. It pulls the pelvis forward in a neutral position. The exercise can be done in several different positions, including kneeling. Start with your hands and knees on the floor. Next, arch your back like a cat and drop your head at the same time. Hold for a count of ten and relax for a count of five. Repeat for one or two minutes at least twice daily.

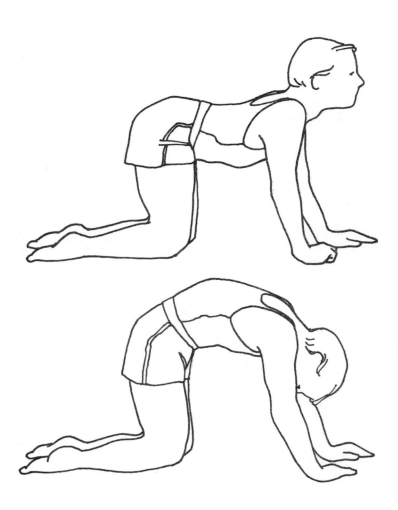

Side-Hip Stretch

This exercise can help to strengthen and limber both the back and the legs. Lie on your side with your legs bent at a 90-degree angle to your body. Place one hand under your head and support your body with the other. As shown below, first straighten the upper leg and then bring it up towards the chin. Return to the original position for a five-count rest, and repeat. When you begin to tire, roll over and repeat the exercise with the other leg.

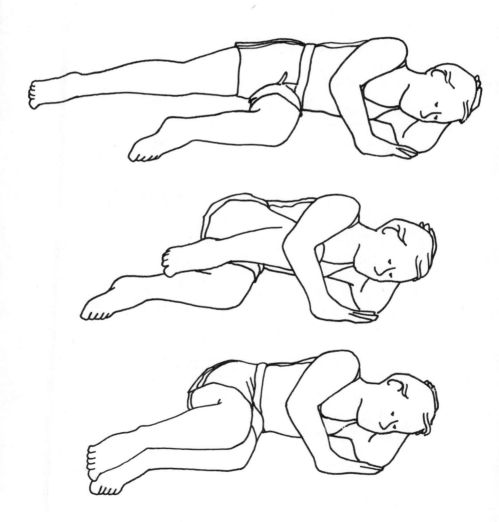

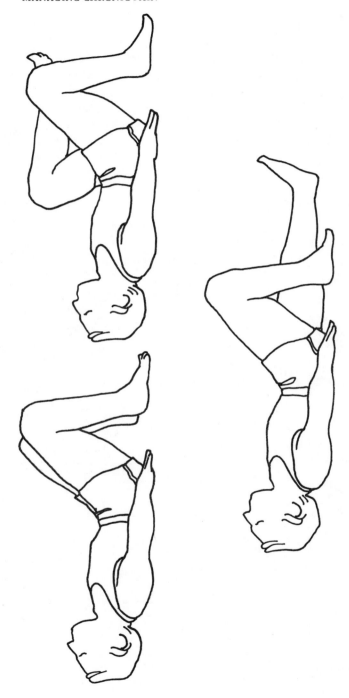

Prone-Hip Stretch

The prone-hip-stretch exercise helps limber tight back and leg muscles. Lie flat on your back with both legs positioned as shown above. Slowly draw one knee towards the chest for five counts and then relax. Repeat with the other knee.

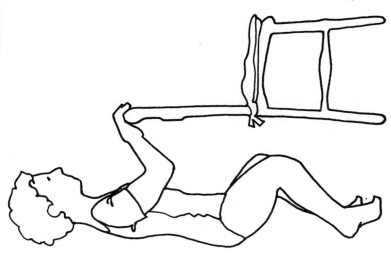

Knee Bends

Knee bends strengthen weak thigh muscles. Weak leg muscles can cause back injuries and pain because people who cannot lift with their legs will compromise and use their backs. Find a table or chair that is about waist-high. Use your hands for balance as you keep your back straight and bend the knees to about a three-quarter squat. Do at least ten knee bends.

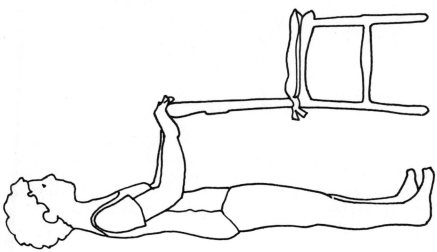

Neck-and-Hip Stretch

This exercise is one that can remedy shortened hip, stomach and neck muscles, which are common causes of back pain. Lie on your back and slowly pull one knee as close to the chest as possible. At the same time, stretch your head down towards your feet as shown. Hold the knee to the chest for a count of five, and repeat with the other knee. Repeat twice daily for two or three minutes.

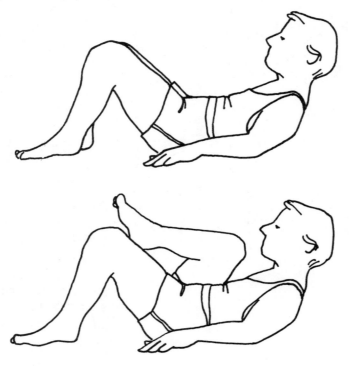

RELIEVING BACK PAIN

In spite of your best efforts at prevention, you may still end up with a backache. Because of its location and structure, the spine is particularly susceptible to injury. Fortunately, up to 90 percent of backaches go away within a few weeks. If your pain does not go away, consult your doctor, who may prescribe one of the following treatments.

Rest

Probably the most important treatment for acute back pain is bed rest. Most backaches are caused by strained muscles that respond well to rest alone. Acute pain is part of our self-defense system, warning us that something is wrong and requires attention. If you injure your back, get in bed and stay there. If your back pain is not improved in three to five days, consult your doctor.

Physical Therapy

Therapeutic heat and cold and massaging the painful area using some type of oil or cream (to reduce friction) can do wonders for an aching back. Massage increases blood flow to muscles and promotes healing. On the day of an injury, ice can be used to control swelling; thereafter, a heating pad or warm-water bottle can bring welcome relief.

Drugs

Prescription drugs may help you rest easier after a back injury, but they will not cure the problem and will have some undesirable side effects. Muscle relaxants, for example, relax you all over and frequently leave you feeling sleepy and drugged. Tranquillizers also produce generalized relaxation and can make you feel groggy. Aspirin is an excellent drug for pain relief and has relatively few negative side effects.

Surgery

Doctors have traditionally sought to relieve back pain through either conservative management, such as bed rest, physical therapy, medication or surgical procedures such as laminectomies, fusions, facet rhizotomies and cordotomies. The most common surgical procedure for back pain involves the removal of a ruptured disc. On carefully selected patients properly screened by a clinical psychologist prior to surgery, the results of surgery are usually good. Overall, however, the results of surgical procedures to relieve back pain are far from acceptable.

A recent article claims that five years after surgery, all but ten percent of back operations have failed to give satisfactory relief of pain to the patient.

If you have back pain, surgery may or may not help. Discuss your treatment options with your doctor. A good doctor will take the time to explain what treatments are available and the likelihood of success. If your doctor is a surgeon and recommends surgery, get a second opinion from a physician who is *not* a surgeon. Don't worry about offending your surgeon. Most surgeons will appreciate your cautious and responsible action. A physiatrist (nonsurgeon specialist in physical medicine and rehabilitation) is an excellent choice to provide a second opinion. If your doctor proceeds with treatment in a cautiously slow and deliberate manner, you probably have a good doctor. Back surgery is serious business and every effort should be made to relieve the pain before scheduling surgery.

Pain Rehabilitation Programs

One of the newer and more innovative approaches to the treatment of pain is the interdisciplinary pain rehabilitation program or "pain clinic" (see Chapter Thirteen). Unfortunately, the concept of pain treatment centers has become quite popular and thus the term can refer to interdisciplinary centers located at major hospitals or to nonlicensed or weakly licensed "practitioners" who offer foot massage and magic for pain relief.

If your back pain has not responded well to traditional medical treatment, a pain rehabilitation program may help. Discuss this with your doctor. Before you invest your time, money and health in a pain treatment program, do some investigation. A good center will have an interdisciplinary staff of doctors and therapists who work with patients on a full-time active basis. Ensure that the center has a clinical psychologist on staff to deal with the psychological aspects of pain. Finally, the schedule should have evening as well as daytime activities. Patients should have both group and individual sessions with the doctors and therapists. Many individuals have been helped at pain rehabilitation programs, and this interdisciplinary concept is becoming increasingly popular.

CHAPTER TEN

Relaxation

Prolonged muscle contraction or muscle tension depletes muscles of oxygen and blood, thereby allowing a buildup of toxins which may result in the sensation we know as pain. In addition, muscle tension requires an expenditure of personal energy, and prolonged tension can result in both needless fatigue and increased susceptibility to physical injury and pain. Your automobile functions only if and when gasoline is burned to move the wheels. There is little difference with your body. Your body also requires fuel to power your muscles and nerves. The name of your "body fuel" is *adenasine triphosphate*—ATP for short, and it is manufactured from the food you eat.

The causes of muscle tension in chronic-pain victims are numerous and varied. Certainly the stress of routine living with children, marriage, work, traffic and finances affects us all. In addition, chronic-pain victims must cope with the frustration, depression and anxiety of an incurable disorder and the physical and psychological stress of continuous pain. Add to that the tension of an impaired life-style and the frustration resulting from a medical system that, until recently, could offer little explanation or relief, and you begin to get a picture of the chronic-pain victim.

Because many chronic-pain victims have suffered increased muscular tension for months and sometimes years, they often lose the natural habit or ability to relax. The typical chronic-pain victim does not know which muscles are tense, cannot accurately judge whether he is relaxed, does not clearly realize that he should relax and does not know how. For many chronic-pain victims, the ability to relax tense, painful muscles and decrease the intensity of pain must be cultivated or acquired anew. It is a skill that has been lost in the confusion and complexity of living with chronic pain. Following popular standards, a patient may be "relaxed" in bed for hours or days; indeed, bed rest is reported by many pain patients as part of their daily routine. However, do not confuse bed rest with muscular relaxation. An individual may "rest" in bed, yet still be anxious and tense during periods of sleep.

If chronically tense muscles aggravate or cause pain, then logically the opposite of tension—relaxation—should decrease pain. Relaxation procedures help manage pain by relieving the anxiety that is usually associated with pain and by allowing an unimpaired blood flow to affected muscles. Relaxation exercises share with EMG biofeedback the same goal of muscular relaxation and usually complement each other. A major difference between the two techniques is that EMG biofeedback targets relaxation of one or two specific muscle groups, while relaxation exercises are targeted towards overall bodily relaxation.

One particularly effective and popular relaxation technique is known as progressive muscular relaxation. It involves having a patient practice simple exercises that mechanically manipulate the skeletal muscles of the entire body into a more relaxed state. Dr. Edmund Jacobson, founder of the Laboratory of Clinical Physiology, Chicago, Illinois, first outlined the principles of progressive muscular relaxation exercises in the early 1900's. The exercises have been modified numerous times since Dr. Jacobson's early publication but still focus on learning to differentiate between muscle tension and deep relaxation. After a patient learns the basic relaxation technique, practice is required to perfect the skill. With serious practice, less time is required to achieve the desired stage of deep muscular relaxation. The technique can then be used to decrease discomfort, to ward off sudden increases in pain associated with increased stress, and to assist with sleep difficulties which may be associated with tension and chronic pain.

LEARNING TO RELAX

Deep muscle relaxation is easy to learn, but the importance of practice cannot be overly emphasized. When practiced on a regular basis, it provides stress reduction, muscle-tension reduction, and time out from pain. For readers interested in learning the technique, the following procedures and techniques are recommended.

Procedure

1. When first learning to relax, a quiet, dimly lit place is an ideal area in which to practice.
2. Lie on your back on a carpeted floor or sit in a comfortable chair. Avoid practicing relaxation exercises in bed since most mattresses do not provide sufficient support.
3. Try to eliminate all other competing thoughts from your mind. Relaxation exercises are intended to relax your body *and* your mind.
4. Focus all attention on the muscle group being tensed.
5. Tense muscle groups on cue. Get in a habit of following the same procedure each time you practice relaxation exercises.
6. Hold the tension and focus all attention on the buildup of tension in every muscle group for six to ten seconds.
7. Release the tension from each muscle group all at once. Do *not* gradually relax a muscle group at the end of six to ten seconds, but instead let the muscle relax suddenly, as if turning off a light switch.
8. After relaxing a muscle group, focus all of your attention on relaxation for twenty to thirty seconds. Concentrate on the different sensation between tension and relaxation.
9. Repeat for each muscle group.
10. Practice relaxation exercises at least twice daily, but the more the better!

Technique (Exercises to be done while you lie on the floor)

1. Make a tight fist and tense the muscles of the forearm of the right arm and hand. Imagine you are holding a golf ball in the palm of the right hand and squeezing it. Relax.
2. Make a tight fist, bending the right arm at the elbow and tensing the muscles of the upper arm. Relax.
3. Make a tight fist and tense the muscles of the forearm of the left arm and hand. Imagine you are holding a golf ball in the palm of the left hand and squeezing it. Relax.

4. Make a tight fist, bending the left arm at the elbow and tensing the muscles of the upper arm. Relax.
5. Tense the muscles of the neck. Push your chin towards your chest, and pulling your head at the same time, lift your head off the floor. Relax.
6. Tense the muscles of your face. Clamp your jaw tightly shut and pull back on the corners of the mouth. Squint your eyes tightly shut and wrinkle your nose. Raise your eyebrows towards your hairline and wrinkle your forehead. Relax.
7. Tense the muscles of your shoulders, chest and back. Take a deep breath and hold it. Now pull the shoulders back and together much like the military attention posture. Relax.
8. Tense the muscle of the abdomen. Take a deep breath and bear down with the stomach muscles. Relax.
9. Tense the muscles of the buttocks and right thigh. Press the back of the right knee down into the floor. Relax.
10. Tense the muscles of the right calf and foot. Bend the foot at the ankle and stretch the toes towards the head. Relax.
11. Tense the muscles of the buttocks and left thigh. Press the back of the left knee down into the floor. Relax.
12. Tense the muscles of the left calf and foot. Bend the foot at the ankle and stretch the toes towards the head. Relax.

When you have completed this exercise, take two to three deep breaths, holding each one for a moment and deeply relaxing yourself as you exhale. Enjoy this relaxed state for a while, breathing regularly and slowly to enhance it. Sometimes imagery may enter your mind when you are deeply relaxed. If pleasant, allow it to continue, and focus on it. When you are ready to end the exercise, count slowly backwards from five to one. Move slowly until fully alert. Remember that the key to managing your pain by achieving deep muscular relaxation is practice!

NOTE: The relaxation exercise described above is but one of many relaxation techniques designed to reduce muscle tension and to manage chronic pain better. It should be noted that while relaxation techniques are very useful, they are not intended as a substitute for professional health care. If you find the technique difficult to learn, if it does not seem to be reducing your tension levels, or if your body feels relaxed but your mind continues to race, seek the assistance of your doctor.

CHAPTER ELEVEN

Cognitive Pain Management

In previous chapters we focused on techniques such as drug treatment, nerve blocks and TENS which disrupt the transmission of pain messages to the brain and on techniques that induce psychophysiological states that are incompatible with pain, such as hypnosis, biofeedback, physical exercise and relaxation. There is another very important component in managing pain which emphasizes changing our thoughts, images and perceptions of pain. The technique is termed cognitive pain management and dates back thousands of years to ancient religious writings.

The basic premise of cognitive pain management is this: What we tell ourselves and how we visualize pain before, during and after the experience has a strong effect on our ability to manage and cope with discomfort. Sound too simple to be true? Then why do many people turn their head when having blood drawn from a finger or arm? Maybe it's because distraction and avoidance of visualizing the needle puncturing the skin seems, somehow, to make the pain less intense. Frequently we prepare ourselves for aversive situations by silently talking to ourselves, visualizing the situation, imagining how it is going to be, and mentally manipulating our thoughts and feelings. Cognitive theory in general is really little more than offering a scientific name and research evidence to document the effectiveness of what most of us have been doing all of our lives.

Cognitive techniques in pain management are based on theories that emphasize the involvement of strong psychological variables in our perception of pain. To illustrate psychological involvement, consider the football player who plays the remainder of a game unaware of a broken foot suffered shortly after the second-half kickoff. Or consider Muhammad Ali who fought a fifteen-round heavyweight fight after suffering a fractured jaw in the fourth round, an injury that generally causes excruciating pain. The excitement and drama of the event, the distraction of the game or fight, and the motivation targeted towards the task at hand combine to defuse the intensity of pain signals.

Cognitive and related theories that emphasize psychological variables in the perception of pain are in direct contrast with specificity theory of pain perception which is still popular in many medical schools. Specificity theory postulates that the intensity of pain is directly proportional to the extent of tissue damage. The theory implies a fixed, straight-through transmission line from any painful part of the body directly to the brain. Specificity theory ignores the overwhelming evidence that pain is not simply a function of the amount of bodily damage alone, but is influenced by attention, anxiety, suggestion, prior conditioning and a host of cognitive variables.

The specificity theory of pain, with its concept of a fixed one-to-one relationship between stimulus and sensation, is not only believed by many researchers to be inaccurate, but also responsible for the expectation in patients and physicians alike that a given form of treatment, in the hands of all doctors, should work for all patients and for all pains. No such treatment has been found, and the complexity and diversity of pain and of patients' and doctors' personalities suggest that it never will. Nevertheless, the idea of the ultimate panacea of total pain relief for everyone pervades our Western culture. The patient who visits a clinic and is told that he must learn to live with his pain usually concludes that the doctor is incompetent and, consequently, the patient visits doctor after doctor in search for the all-encompassing, perfect pain-control method. The patients who have visited lists of doctors and spent thousands of dollars for health care are, in large part, products of our Western all-or-nothing, pill-popping ethos, which promises instant, total pain relief—if not today, then tomorrow.

Health care practitioners must also accept a portion of the blame for this state of affairs, and their training in specificity concepts underlies it. One pain, one cause—eliminate the cause by an operation or a drug and the pain should vanish. This works often enough for acute pain. Chronic pain, however, which generally has multiple determinants, is an entirely different story. Treatment may sometimes enhance rather than diminish pain, which may lead to further treatment that may make the patient worse. It is not that uncommon to see a patient crippled with back pain, who has undergone several disc operations and other types of surgery for pain relief, and who finally is turned over to a psychologist or psychiatrist. The so-called cause of pain has been eliminated and if the patient is still in pain, he is by definition (in terms of specificity theory), a malingerer or neurotic. Small wonder that by this time the patient is depressed, resentful, anxious and attentive only to his pain. It is a fundamental fact in the field of pain that some patients will suffer pain for the rest of their lives. In such cases, the most effective therapy may be to teach them to live with their pain, to carry on productive lives in spite of it.

Cognitive Techniques: A Novel Approach

Our past failures in managing pain may be due to concentrating efforts on the physiology of pain while ignoring the psychology of pain. Many doctors today realize that pain has both physical and psychological components, and attending to one while ignoring the other is setting the stage for failure.

A number of cognitive management techniques have been suggested to help those patients whose pain persists despite the best efforts of modern medicine. One of the more interesting and innovative cognitive techniques was recently reported by Dr. Ira D. Turkat and Dr. R. Bruce Craft.* (Dr. Turkat is presently director of the clinical psychology program of the Diabetes Research and Training Center at Vanderbilt University, Nashville, Tennessee. Dr. Craft is with the Veterans Administration Hospital in Augusta, Georgia.) Their three-phase program is based on the following rationale: Pain responses can be learned; cognitive interpretation of pain may affect the pain experience, making the

---

* "Behavioral Modification of Pain: A Clinical Innovation," *Behavioral Medicine*, May 1980, p. 33–35. Excerpts from this publication regarding cognitive management techniques appear on pgs. 108–111.

pain more or less severe; psychological pain control is a skill like any other skill; and expectancy for improvement must be realistic. A typical rationale may be presented to the patient as follows:

How we respond to pain is very often learned. For example, a professional boxer learns not to show the pain he experiences while in the boxing ring. However, you and I have learned to express our pain when we experience these sensations. Because we learn to experience pain in certain ways, we can also learn to experience it in new ways. Thus, I would like to help you learn to experience your pain in a new way.

Once the patient understands and agrees that pain experiences can also be learned, the following information is carefully explained to the patient:

As you are probably aware, the way in which you experience pain very often depends on how you interpret the pain. For example, if you stub your toe and focus intensely on the pain sensations, it appears to be more painful than when you focus on something else, trying to ignore the pain. Thus, by teaching you a different way to interpret pain, you may be able to learn to control your pain.

Following the patient's acknowledgement that cognitive interpretation of pain may be a very important aspect of learning how to best control chronic pain, the following information is presented:

It is important to realize that learning to control pain is a skill like any other. Like learning to swim or drive a car, the more you practice the skill, the better you will be at it. Thus, in the pain-control program you will be requested to practice the pain-control strategy quite frequently. You will find that the more you practice, the better you will be at using the strategy. You may find that the pain-control strategy may completely eliminate the pain. You may find that the strategy may not help very much. I cannot guarantee that your pain problem will be completely resolved. However, I can say that the more you practice the pain-control strategy, the better you will be at using the strategy.

Phase I

Following a baseline period during which information is gathered on each patient's pain intensity, the number of hours each day that the victims experience pain, and the number of milligrams of pain medication that each patient takes daily, the following written instructions are circulated:

In order for you to become good at controlling pain, you must practice the pain-control strategy every day. It has been our experience that 15-minute practice sessions, once in the morning and once in the evening, are very helpful in learning to control pain.

The first phase in learning how to control pain involves practicing the pain-control strategy on a part of the body that is not a pain problem for you. This is because it is easier to learn the strategy on a nonpainful area than on a painful area. Once you become very skilled at controlling sensations in the nonpainful area, then it becomes easier to apply the strategy to a painful area.

Now we are ready to learn the pain-control strategy. It is easy to learn because all that it requires is imagination and concentration. The more you practice the strategy, the better you will become at it.

First, pick a part of the body that is not a pain problem for you. If possible, try using your right hand to practice the strategy. If not, pick another body part with which to practice the strategy. Close your eyes and concentrate very hard on imagining this body part as having no sensation at all. You might imagine the body part as being completely without feeling as if it were made of rubber. Just describe in your mind how this body part has no feeling in it, is completely dead, no feeling whatsoever, like it's made of hard rubber. Just continue concentrating on this body part as having no feeling at all. You might imagine looking at the body part and notice that it looks like hard rubber. Use whatever thoughts you can think of to imagine the body part as having no sensation at all. Practice the strategy over and over again.

It is important at this phase that you use the same body part every day to practice the strategy with. Do not attempt to use the strategy on the painful body part yet. This will be done later on when you have become very skilled in using the strategy. This decision will be made jointly by you and your therapist.

Phase II

The second phase of the pain-control program is initiated when the patient reports being able to imagine clearly pain insensitivity in a nonpainful body part. This is determined by having the patient rate his or her ability to imagine pain insensitivity on a scale from zero to ten (ten equals complete insensitivity) and able to report ten for seven successive days. Upon reaching this criterion, the following information is presented:

> Now that you have learned to experience no sensation at all in a body part which is not a pain problem for you, such as your right hand, it is important to practice the pain-control strategy in a way that will help you with your pain problem. In order to do this effectively, you must continue to practice the strategy, but in a different way.

> The next step in learning to control pain involves the following procedure: Take the nonpainful body part that you have practiced the pain-control strategy on and place it on top of the painful body part. Imagine the nonpainful body part as being completely without sensation but do *not* try to imagine the painful areas as insensitive. Focus *only* on the nonpainful body part and imagine it as being completely without feeling, even though it is placed on top of the painful area. Remember, concentrate only on the nonpainful body part and ignore the painful body part.

> Learning to experience the nonpainful body part as if it were without feeling *while* it is placed on top of the painful body part requires a good deal of practice. Thus, it is important that you continue to practice the strategy at least twice a day for 15 minutes per practice session. You may notice that it may take you more time to master this skill than in the first phase of the pain-control program. It may even take less time. In any event, you must practice the strategy quite often in order to become good at it.

> After practicing the strategy for a period of time, you may notice that the painful body part is also beginning to feel as if it has no sensation, even though you are only concentrating on the nonpainful area. This is quite common and is part of the skill-learning process. Remember, do *not* attempt to use the strategy on your painful area yet. This will be done later on when you

have become very skilled in using Phase II of the pain-control strategy. This decision will be made jointly by both you and your therapist.

Phase III

Phase III, the final phase of the cognitive-treatment program, is initiated when the patient reaches a criterion similar to that specified in Phase II. In this phase the patient learns to apply the principles of pain control to the painful body area:

Now that you have learned to experience no sensation at all in a body part which is not a pain problem for you, while it is placed on top of the painful body part, it is time for you to take the strategy one step further so that you may use it to control pain. This next step is the final phase of the pain-control program. Once you have mastered this skill, by continuous practice, you will be able to apply the strategy to other parts that may become a pain problem for you.

Instead of focusing on a nonpainful part as being completely without feeling, apply the pain-control strategy to the painful area *only*. Concentrate on imagining the painful body part as if it had no feeling whatsoever—like hard rubber—no sensation at all. Practice the strategy over and over again.

It is important that you continue to practice the strategy at least twice per day and more if necessary. The more you practice, the better you will be at controlling your pain.

HINTS FOR COGNITIVE PAIN CONTROL

It is important to recognize that with training and practice, cognitive pain-management techniques can be powerful and effective weapons in the battle against pain. Needless to say, cognitive techniques are not a "cure-all" and do not imply that pain is "all in your head." When properly used, however, cognitive strategies can be successfully employed to reduce the intensity, frequency and duration of discomfort and suffering, and the techniques are readily available to each of us. All that is required is a decision to take personal responsibility and active control of your pain, to work as a "partner" with your doctor rather than presenting yourself as a passive recipient of medical care to doctor after doctor. This decision, combined with a great deal of practice, can help set you on the track toward controlling your pain, rather than have your pain control you! Here are some hints:

1. Distraction. Concentration is a skill that can be developed with practice in much the same way that skills in golf, cooking, swimming or playing tennis can be sharpened. Intense concentration on something other than pain will block the discomfort from consciousness. Your mind, which can only fully concentrate on one thought or object at a time, will be distracted from the perception of pain. Dentists have long used distraction as a pain-management technique by placing the dental chair in a position that looks out a window or by placing a picture on a wall in front of the patient. Distraction techniques that may work for you include mental arithmetic problems such as counting backwards by threes from one hundred, or even sexual fantasies!

2. Stopping Negative Self-Talk. Most of us spend a good portion of every day "talking to ourselves." Silent internal dialogue, or self-talk, is a way of planning and organizing our thoughts and feelings. Since pain is a negative sensation, our self-talk about thoughts and feelings of pain is also usually negative. Negative self-talk is associated with anxiety and increased pain. It has not occurred to most people that internal statements, or self-talk, can be managed and controlled with practice, thereby reducing discomfort and pain.

3. Positive Thinking. A change from negative self-talk to positive thinking can have a significant effect on the pain you experience. Just as negative self-talk is associated with anxiety and increased pain, positive thinking is associated with and reinforces confidence, relaxation and equanimity. It requires determination and practice, but the results can be a dramatic reduction in pain intensity.

4. Controlling Anxiety. It has been noted throughout this text that anxiety and associated muscle tension increase pain levels, while relaxation and calm are associated with decreased pain intensity. Mental and physiological calm are required for effective pain control. To control anxiety, practice the progressive relaxation exercises outlined in Chapter Ten until you can achieve a state of deep muscular and mental relaxation within minutes. In addition, try wearing a rubber band around your wrist as a reminder to pause periodically throughout the day, slowly count backwards from ten to zero, take a deep breath, and *relax*!

5. Concentrating on Abilities, Not Disabilities. One of the many complexities associated with chronic pain is that patients naturally focus on activities that were once a part of their lives, and now believed impossible because of pain. Such activities may include recreational and vocational interests. Understandably, many chronic-pain patients concentrate on activities they can no longer do, and pain becomes the center of their lives. To avoid the increased pain and misery such thinking creates, spend time identifying and perfecting your abilities. If you can no longer participate in football, how about softball? If you can no longer perform a job that requires sitting eight hours each day, how about a job that involves walking? Chronic pain is *not* a totally disabling disorder. Some concentration and practice on your abilities rather than your disabilities will prove this to be true!

Modifying Pain
Behavior

Pain may be considered to be a subjective internal sensation, but it is also partly behavior which is communicated to
those around us in a variety of ways. We may moan, grimace,
talk about the quality and location of discomfort, limp and move
in a guarded manner, take medications, and spend excessive
amounts of time resting or in bed. We look for assistance and
sympathy from family, friends, employers, doctors and acquain-
tances. These are examples of pain behaviors which inform
others that we are in distress. Without some form of pain communication, intentional or otherwise, no one would know that
we were in discomfort, since pain cannot be seen except in the
pain behaviors we exhibit.

Our family, friends and doctors usually react to pain behaviors in the direction of active assistance as well as solicitous-
ness and special concern. This concern is considered by some
researchers to be of both an amateur (responses of family and
friends) and professional (doctors and nurses) nature. In both
cases the special attention afforded the patient in distress is
pain-contingent. In other words, no communication of pain, no
special attention. Nevertheless, both amateur and professional
concern and attention are usually helpful, at least in acute pain,
since the responses of others often leads to some reduction in
our level of distress. The solicitous spouse may not reduce our
intensity of pain, but his or her attention and care may help
reduce our fear. If the spouse steps in to take over the tasks
which aggravate our pain, he or she has been even more helpful.
Whatever the case, there is likely to be pain-contingent attention

114

and, associated with it, some relief. The attention itself usually has reinforcing properties in that it is positive and enjoyable. When attention is associated with some relief in our distress, the reinforcing properties can be expected to increase.

The likelihood of relief and reinforcement is even greater in the case of professional attention in response to pain behaviors. The probable impact of professional pain-contingent attention is enhanced yet further by the prestige of the professional. The special and focussed attention of a doctor, for example, is usually more socially reinforcing to most of us than the attention of most other persons encountered in a typical day.

So here we have potentially potent amateur and professional reinforcement which occurs, to some degree, contingent upon the display and communication of pain behaviors. As a result, we systematically and naturally "learn" to elicit helping, solicitous responses from others by temporarily adopting a "sick role" and by communicating pain behaviors.

Such a natural situation may potentially complicate many cases of chronic pain. Operant psychology tells us that we tend to act in ways to best shape the future to our advantage. In other words, "we learn by noticing what effects our actions and behaviors have on the world and build up patterns of repetitive behavior—strategies—that will maximize positive and minimize negative effects in the future."* For instance, after receiving a speeding ticket, most of us try to stay within the speed limit since speeding increases our chances of further negative effects.

Operant psychology is particularly applicable to pain. After suffering a neck injury that landed us in bed for a week or two, we're likely to modify our behavior in an effort to guard against a recurrence of the injury. Perhaps we move about guardedly, undergo corrective surgery, take analgesic medication, stay off our feet as much as possible, possibly avoid the physical exertion of work by staying home, all the while communicating our discomfort and vulnerability to others so we can avoid situations that might require moving and acting in a way that increases our risk of further injury.

If our pain behaviors succeed and the pain gradually diminishes, we have effectively modified our behavior to adjust to

Mastering Pain, p. 179.

the temporary disruption of pain. As the pain subsides, we gradually get back into our regular pattern of behavior, possibly exercising a bit more caution when lifting or straining, but generally we're our old selves again.

But what happens if our pain behaviors are not successful and our pain is not eliminated? What if the best efforts of our doctors do not result in decreased suffering, and every movement continues to result in pain? What if our painkilling drugs prove ineffective and we take ever-stronger medication, with the mental confusion, nausea and cognitive dulling associated with high-powered narcotic use a result? What if our search for relief takes us back to the operating room, but again, no relief?

Then the stage is set for the potential development of a chronic-pain syndrome. Our experience tells us that natural coping behaviors should work towards the resolution of our discomfort. They are tried-and-true and have always worked before. Now, however, they do not work, the pain persists or even increases, and we are caught unprepared in a novel situation. Panic sets in. Rather than adopting a new strategy to deal with the pain, we try to force those behaviors which have always worked for us in the past. We desperately call on them to work again. We visit another doctor and then another. We swallow more and stronger pills, desperately searching for a cure. Experience tells us to persist in our usual behaviors targeted towards pain relief.

Consider the hypothetical case of John, 43, who injured himself when he tripped and fell while carrying a toolbox at work. John was immediately taken to the emergency room of a local hospital, where he complained of pain in the lower back and down the right leg. X rays were taken and he was thoroughly examined by both an emergency-room physician and an orthopedic surgeon. Both the X rays and physical examinations were normal, and he was sent home with instructions from the surgeon to stay in bed for one week, take the pain-pills he was given, and return for an office visit in one week.

John was showered with attention and care the following week by his concerned wife, children and colleagues at work. Even the owner of the plant sent flowers and telephoned to inquire about his health. John returned to his doctor at the appointed time, limping, moaning and complaining of severe pain.

The doctor hospitalized John and increased the strength of medication. John tried to get out of bed to go to the bathroom, but the pain was excruciating. Several visitors assisted him to the bathroom while his wife, generally inattentive and aloof prior to the injury, cried softly from the corner of the room. A myelogram was performed which turned out negative. John stayed in bed and hurt, a strained look of anguish and distress on his face, while a representative of the employer's insurance company sympathized and completed the necessary paperwork to start financial compensation.

John continued to be in pain one month later, and two months later his health was the same. Most days are now spent going to a new doctor or hobbling around the backyard. Occasionally he will drive down to his former place of employment, limp through the warehouse, grimace as he supports himself with a cane, stop every few feet to sit and rest, and talk about the horror of his constant pain to anyone who will listen. His wife and friends listen, as does a different doctor every few weeks. John never tries a different approach; he is tightly webbed in the trap of chronic pain. There is no hope for change, until John decides to change.

When normal pain behaviors fail to bring relief, as they did with John, what is needed is new pain behavior, new attempts to learn an effective means of managing pain. We are creatures of habit, and adopting a totally new approach to dealing with pain does not come easily for most of us. In addition, while relief from pain does not come from old patterns of behavior, it does bring other positive consequences: attention and concern from others, euphoria from narcotic drugs, a break from the daily work grind, and maybe even financial compensation from employers and insurance companies for not being able to work. These positive consequences may outweigh the disadvantage of continued pain, thereby reinforcing and exacerbating chronic-pain behavior.

If you feel the above description is relevant to your pain, the solution is clear: Break the strong connection between pain behavior and its positive consequences. When this is accomplished, shift the positive consequences to reinforce and support "well behavior". This is best accomplished in many cases in an environment such as an inpatient chronic-pain program where medications, attention, contingencies and reinforcements can be controlled. In the following chapter on pain clinics, a description of a Chronic Pain Rehabilitation Program will outline how this is accomplished. In less severe cases, a determined effort on your part and the active assistance of your family and doctor can often produce significant results. The following information is presented as a general guide for you and your family. Discuss these hints with your family and your doctor and, with their approval and assistance, give it a try.

Modifying Your Pain Behavior

Even when pain lingers on and on, there are ways of making yourself feel better. Here are some hints that have worked for many people. Your doctor can help you tailor the program to your specific needs. Keep the hints handy as a reminder of the general principles. The goals of the program are to:

1. Reduce the amount of medication you are taking or eliminate it altogether.
2. Reduce your pain.
3. Increase your activity level.
4. Get you back to work.

To meet these program goals, try these five suggestions:

1. *Realize that although others can try to help, only you can make yourself feel better.* Your doctor, family and friends can give you advice and support, but you have to assume responsibility for relieving your pain and taking an active role in the management of your problem.
2. *Gradually decrease the amount of medication you take.* Pain relievers rarely help chronic pain. After you have taken a pain medication for a long time, your body develops tolerance, so the drug no longer provides relief. It may make you feel better, but this is because your body has become dependent on the medication. Due to this dependence, your doctor will not stop the medication abruptly. He will slowly reduce the amount of medication you take, giving your body a chance to get used to being without it.
3. *Focus on your activities rather than your pain.* Try to stop thinking and talking about how much you hurt; it will only

make you feel worse. Becoming more active and thinking and talking about what you're doing will help take your mind off your pain.

4. *Gradually increase your level of activity.* Unless your doctor has a reason to advise against it, activity is not harmful! Acute pain, like that from a twisted ankle, is a protective and warning signal that rest is needed. However, when pain has continued for several months, the presence of pain does not necessarily mean something bad will happen if you gradually increase your level of physical activity.

5. *Go back to work.* Working is good for us and especially good for chronic-pain victims. Working is an excellent example of well behavior. Working will also give you a good reason to get up and get dressed each morning and will help keep you active. Chronic pain is seldom a totally disabling disorder.

Helping the Family Member with Chronic Pain

With the assistance of your doctor, your relative or friend who has a chronic-pain problem may benefit from efforts to modify his or her pain behavior. The goals of this program are to reduce pain, cut down the amount of medication needed for pain, increase his physical activity level, and decrease the communication of pain. In order for your friend or family member to be successful, he will need your help, as follows:

1. *Do not talk about pain.* When someone talks about his pain, he is going to feel worse. Try these suggestions:
   (a) When he starts talking about his pain, let him finish the statement, but try to divert his attention by introducing a new subject when he pauses for breath.
   (b) When he talks about his pain, break eye contact.
   (c) Avoid asking about his pain. Instead, focus on his activities. For instance, when you return from work or shopping, don't ask how he feels, but ask what he did while you were gone.

2. *Help your friend or relative increase his activity level. Activity is not harmful, even when it hurts.* Only acute pain, such as that due to a strain or sprain, requires rest. After pain has continued for several months, the presence of pain upon movement usually means the part is stiff and weak from

lack of use. As the muscles get back into shape, the pain will most likely diminish.

Your doctor can help set a realistic exercise goal for you. The amount of activity should increase a little every two or three days. After the activity level goes up, the pain level will probably go down. Many people who follow this program resume an active life even if the pain persists. Your role is to do the following:

1. Give encouragement by praising increases in activity and encouraging him when he seems to be faltering.
2. Plan interesting activities both in and out of the home.
3. Avoid reinforcing or rewarding him by responding to complaints of pain.

CHAPTER THIRTEEN

The Pain Clinics—
What They Can
Do for You

What is a pain clinic? Unfortunately, just about any place that wants to call itself one. There has been a pain-clinic explosion in the United States since 1976, at which time a survey counted seventeen such clinics. No one is sure how many pain treatment programs exist today, but educated guesses range from five hundred to more than one thousand. Today pain clinics run the range from nonlicensed or weakly licensed "quacks" to interdisciplinary programs involving clinical psychologists, physiatrists, neurosurgeons, orthopedic surgeons, anesthesiologists, occupational therapists, recreational therapists, physical therapists, biofeedback technicians, vocational counselors, rehabilitation nurses and others.

Interdisciplinary pain-treatment programs are undoubtedly the "state of the art." No one of the many treatment techniques described in this book is as likely to assist in the control of your pain as is a combination of therapies. Chronic pain is a multifaceted problem, and effective management is best accomplished with an interdisciplinary approach to treatment. Interdisciplinary means that a number of different doctors and therapists representing a variety of specialties work together *with* the patient towards successful pain control. Estimates are that approximately thirty-five to forty programs in the United States fit the description of an interdisciplinary pain program. Chronic pain is far more complex than the discomfort per se. In addition to pain, many chronic-pain victims suffer disrupted marital and family relationships, disability, loss of or decreased income, drug addiction or dependence, depression and anxiety, deconditioned physical states and other associated physical and psychological problems. In this age of the "superspecialists," an interdisciplinary team approach assures that all aspects of chronic pain will receive professional attention.

It is nearly impossible to describe what may be expected from treatment offered at a pain clinic or program. Pain treatment centers may be inpatient or outpatient, function with no doctors or a staff of specialists, have a wide-ranging cost span for a six-week hospitalization, administer one type of treatment or function as an interdisciplinary team, accept every patient referred or intensively screen out two of every three patients evaluated as "inappropriate," and so on. A solution to describing such a variety of programs is to describe one program. As Director of an interdisciplinary Chronic Pain Rehabilitation Program, the general description that I present is limited to the pain program of the Greenville, South Carolina Hospital System.

Chronic Pain Rehabilitation Program

The Chronic Pain Rehabilitation Program is designed for selected patients who have suffered persisting pain for longer than six months without satisfactory response to traditional medical treatment. The "average" pain patient may be described as suffering from low-back and/or neck pain as the result of an injury (although other types of pain are treated), unemployed or physically and/or psychologically disabled, having undergone as many as seven major operations for pain relief, habituated or dependent on narcotic medication, experiencing serious and significant depression, demonstrating a loss of interest in physical, vocational and social activities, and suffering a breakdown in family and interpersonal relationships.

The Chronic Pain Rehabilitation Program is designed to counteract the disabling effects of chronic pain. Treatment is interdisciplinary and comprehensive as each therapy interrelates during the average 21- to 28-day inpatient hospitalization. The primary treatment team includes a clinical psychologist/ behavioral medicine specialist, physiatrist (physician who specializes in physical medicine), physical therapist, occupational therapist, recreational therapist, social worker, vocational rehabilitation counselor and nursing. Consultants representing neurosurgery, orthopedic surgery, general and thoracic surgery, and psychiatry offer specialized services as needed.

Treatment in the Chronic Pain Rehabilitation Program is not the passive servicing of sick persons found in general hospitals, but is active, goal-oriented, and directive (Table 13–1). Treatment rewards "wellness" and independence as the patient and staff actively work towards positive changes in the patient's physical and psychological life-style. The endless cycle of drugs, doctors, surgeries, suffering and disability is broken as the patient is taught more effective means of pain control and, as a result, adopts a more active, productive and independent style of living. The goals of the Chronic Pain Rehabilitation Program are:

1. Reduction of pain behavior in each patient.
2. Establishment and maintenance of effective well behavior.
3. Increase in frequency and extent of physical exercise and activity.
4. Reduction or elimination of medication intake.
5. Rearrangement of responses to both pain and well behavior by family and significant others (e.g., friends, employer, etc.).
6. Reduction of excessive health care utilization.
7. Reduction of disability.
8. Return to work force (when appropriate).

While admission to some pain treatment centers is almost automatic, patients referred to the Chronic Pain Rehabilitation Program are carefully evaluated and screened prior to acceptance. Preadmission evaluations involve comprehensive physical and psychological examinations, completion of questionnaires (Table 13–2), and evaluations by physical, occupational and recreational therapists as well as social workers. An offer of acceptance to the pain program is contingent, in part, on the results of the preadmission evaluation and a belief by staff members that the patient is truly motivated and determined to learn to manage his pain. As the result of this and other stringent criteria, approximately one of every three patients evaluated is offered program admission. By concentrating on quality rather than quantity, the intensive efforts required to reverse the downward spiral of chronic-pain disability can be fully extended to every patient.

TABLE 13-1: DAILY PATIENT SCHEDULE

Time	Monday	Tuesday	Wednesday	Thursday	Friday	Saturday	Sunday
7:30	Breakfast—Cafeteria	Breakfast—Cafeteria	Breakfast—Cafeteria	Breakfast—Cafeteria	Breakfast—Cafeteria	Breakfast—Cafeteria	Breakfast—Cafeteria
8:00	Self and Room Care	Self and Room Care	Self and Room Care	Self and Room Care	Self and Room Care	Self and Room Care	Self and Room Care
8:30						Individual Exercise	Individual Exercise
9:00	Exercise Class	Exercise Class	Exercise Class	Exercise Class	Exercise Class		
9:30	Relaxation Class	Relaxation Class	Relaxation Class	Relaxation Class	Relaxation Class		Leisure Time/Church
10:00	R.T.	R.T.	R.T.	R.T.	R.T.	Leisure Time	
10:30							
11:00	Group Therapy	Leisure Time	Group Therapy	Leisure Time	Group Therapy	R.T.	R.T.
11:30							
12:00	Lunch	O.T. and Lunch	Lunch	O.T. and Lunch	Lunch	Lunch	Lunch
12:30							
1:00	O.T.		O.T.		O.T.	P.T.	
1:30							Leisure-Visiting
2:00	Pain School—Psychology	Pain School—Nursing	Pain School—P.T.	Pain School—Social Services	Pain School—O.T.	Leisure-Visiting	
2:30							
3:00	P.T.	P.T.	P.T.	P.T.	Vocational Rehabilitation		
3:30							
4:00	R.T.		R.T.		R.T.	R.T.	R.T.
4:30					Leisure-Visiting	Leisure-Visiting	Leisure-Visiting
5:00			Dinner	Leisure Time	Individual Psychology Rounds		
5:30							
6:00		Pain Group Meeting with Families			Visiting		Leisure Time
6:30	R.T.		R.T.	R.T.			
7:00	Visiting	Visiting	Visiting	Visiting			
7:30							
8:00							

R.T. = Recreational Therapy; O.T. = Occupational Therapy; P.T. = Physical Therapy

Behavior Modification

One of the major differences between the Chronic Pain Re-habilitation Program and an acute-care treatment facility is that the structure of the pain-program therapies is geared towards encouraging well behavior and discouraging pain behavior. An operant conditioning environment is employed whereby the con-sequences of pain behaviors are modified in such a way as to neutralize their positive reinforcing value. For example, patients are not to talk about their pain except at designated times, and independence in self-care is emphasized. In fact, patients are treated more as students or athletes in training than as traditional hospital patients. Patients are expected to work hard and be involved in their individualized pain management program.

Physical, Occupational and Recreational Therapies

Chronic-pain problems frequently result from patients being in poor physical condition. Many patients become bedridden or greatly reduce their physical activities for prolonged periods fol-lowing a painful injury. Movements are guarded and minimal with postural impairment often resulting from extended favoring of an affected body part. One important function of physical, occupational and recreational therapists is to gradually exercise and strengthen patients' muscles and joints in a graduated, phys-ical conditioning program. Group and individual exercise ses-sions are scheduled daily to increase range of motion and in-crease endurance. Therapists also use specific pain-reducing treatments such as TENS, biofeedback, cryotherapy, hydro-therapy and ultrasound on an "as needed" individual basis.

Psychotherapy

The intensity of pain is a subjective perception strongly in-fluenced by numerous psychological variables. Consider "Farmer Brown" who, while casually walking across a pasture, accidentally steps in a hole and sprains his ankle. He sits in the grass a long while in intense pain until he struggles to his feet and slowly hobbles towards the farmhouse. He hears an unnerving sound, immediately stops and whirls around to see a huge bull charging towards him. Farmer Brown reacts instantly, running towards the fence and the safety of the other side with lightning quickness, the agony of the sprained ankle forgotten in the overwhelming urgency of the stampeding bull. When safely outside the fenced pasture and with the raging bull turned back, the ankle begins to throb and ache once again, and Farmer Brown agonizingly hobbles towards home.

In the Chronic Pain Rehabilitation Program, patients are taught to manipulate psychological variables by learning to use the most powerful pain-control agent known to man—the human mind. In daily group and individual therapy sessions, patients are instructed in how best to relax, how to use cognitive management techniques by focussing their concentration on topics other than pain, how to redirect thinking towards more positive thoughts, and how to avoid using pain behavior as an escape. Special emphasis is centered on managing the anxiety and depression so often closely associated with chronic pain. In group and individual psychotherapy, patients learn they have two choices: They can either learn to control their pain or allow their pain to control them.

Family Counseling

When patients are admitted to the Chronic Pain Rehabilitation Program, their families, in essence, are admitted as well. Simply stated, it is difficult to treat one without treating the other, since pain and disability become such major components in the lives of most patients *and* their families. In addition, family members often determine the ultimate success of our program, based on how well they encourage well behavior and adhere to the principles of pain management once the patient is discharged. Family and patient group therapy sessions are scheduled weekly, and family members are updated on the patient's progress in the pain program. They are also taught methods to ensure the maintenance of treatment gains once the patient is discharged.

Drug Detoxification

Most chronic-pain patients have been treated extensively with multiple tranquillizers, sedatives, narcotics and synthetic pain relievers, frequently leading to tolerance and dependence. These drugs can also lead to personality changes, which may hinder efforts to return patients to a normal life-style. One of the goals of the Chronic Pain Rehabilitation Program is to slowly, but steadily, reduce drug dependence and consumption. This is accomplished by giving pain medications in a "pain cocktail." A pain cocktail involves administering medications in a liquid vehicle which masks color and taste. The liquid medicine, usually masked with cherry syrup, is then administered on a time-contingent basis rather than a PRN or "as needed" basis. Over time, the amount of active medication ingredients is reduced gradually to allow the patient time to adjust to decreased medication intake.

The ultimate goal of all comprehensive pain-control programs is to return you to as active, productive and meaningful a life as possible. This may mean helping you return to work in your original occupation or assist in retraining for new employment. It also means helping you to control your pain so that, if it cannot be totally eliminated, you can learn to manage it and minimize the disruptive effects on your life. As previously mentioned, the choice is yours—you can learn to control your pain or allow the pain to control you.

TABLE 13-2
CHRONIC-PAIN REHABILITATION PROGRAM PAIN EVALUATION: PATIENT FORM

1. Indicate your name, address, phone number, sex, date of birth and Social Security number.
2. Give the name and address of the physician who referred you.
3. Specify your religion, noting denomination.
4. Specify to which racial group you belong.
5. Indicate your country of birth, as well as that of your parents.
6. Highest grade of school completed: Less than 8th grade; completed 8th grade; did not complete high school; completed high school; technical or business school; some college; completed college; graduate or professional school.

7. Do you live alone; with spouse; with children; with others (roommate, etc.); with brothers and/or sisters; or with other relatives? If you live with other relatives, specify.
8. Note current marital status. If married, separated, divorced or widowed, how long?
9. If married, would you describe your marriage as very satisfactory; satisfactory; tolerable or intolerable?
10. Causes of marital problems and conflicts: money; children; parents and/or in-laws; work situation; personality differences; sexual problems; physical illnesses; religion; my pain.
11. Weekly family income from all sources: less than $100; $101–$200; $201–$300; $301–$400; over $401.
12. Indicate number of individuals supported on family income.
13. Indicate all sources of income: salary; retirement; pension; Social Security; personal disability insurance; investments; compensation; Social Security disability; other (describe).
14. If married, what is your spouse's occupation? (Be specific.)
15. The following questions relate to your employment, which includes work as a housewife. Please answer all questions that apply to you:
    (A) At what age did you begin working?
    (B) How many jobs have you had since you first began working?
    (C) What is your specific occupation? Briefly describe what you do.
    (D) Are you presently employed full-time, part-time, or as a housewife? If employed, how long?
    (E) If you are unemployed or employed part-time, is this due to your present pain condition?
    (F) How long have you been working in your last job? If unemployed, retired or disabled, how long?
    (G) Do you enjoy your work all the time; most of the time; some of the time; rarely or not at all?
    (H) Does your work provide you with a feeling of satisfaction all of the time; most of the time; some of the time; rarely or not at all?
    (I) In general, before your injury, did your employer treat you fairly?
16. If your present pain condition was caused by your job or occurred while on the job or was due to an accident, please answer the following:
    (A) Was your employer helpful and understanding of your problem?

(B) Do you believe he has been fair in his treatment of you since you have been sick/injured?

(C) Have you received compensation (money) for your injury?

(D) If you have received compensation, do you feel it has been adequate?

(E) Are you bringing suit (suing) because of your injury?

(F) Have you already had to sue to get compensation?

(G) Have you tried to return to work?

(H) Did your employer allow you to return?

(I) Do you think you can work full-time, part-time or not at all at your regular job?

(J) Compared to your ability to do your job before your injury, can you now do as much as before; less than before; much less than before or can't do the job at all?

17. Comparing your condition before you had pain with your present condition, please answer the questions below:

(A) My *desire* for social activities remains about the same as before; somewhat less than before; very much less than before; no desire for social activities.

(B) My *ability* to engage in social activities remains about the same as before; is somewhat less than before; is very much less than before; I no longer have the ability.

(C) My *desire* for hobbies and recreational interests remains about the same as before; is somewhat less than before; is very much less than before; no desire.

(D) My *ability* to engage in hobbies and recreational activities remains about the same as before; is somewhat less than before; is very much less than before; I no longer have the ability.

(E) My *desire* for sexual activities remains about the same as before; is somewhat less than before; is very much less than before; no desire for sexual relations.

(F) My *ability* to engage in sexual activities remains about the same as before; is somewhat less than before; is very much less than before; I no longer have the ability.

18. Have you ever had psychological or psychiatric treatment or evaluation for any condition or problem? If yes, give condition of most recent treatment.

19. Do you feel you are helpless to change your present condition? Never; some of the time; most of the time; all of the time.

20. Do you feel your present condition is hopeless? Never; some of the time; most of the time; all of the time.

21. Aside from your pain problem, are you frequently ill?
22. Are you frequently confined to bed because of poor health, other than because of pain?
23. Do others consider you a sickly person?
24. Do you consider yourself to be a sickly person?
25. Do you come from a sickly family?
26. Was any member of your family disabled due to a pain problem?
27. Does it seem that suffering is your way of life? Never; sometimes; most of the time; always feel that way.
28. Are you often miserable and unhappy?
    (A) Is your appetite good or poor?
    (B) Do you have crying spells or feel like it?
    (C) Are you more irritable than usual?
29. The following frequently increase or decrease chronic pain. Choose which of the following apply to you and your pain:

Stimulants (coffee, etc.)	Lying down
Liquor	Sitting
Eating	Driving
Heat	Distraction (TV, etc.)
Cold	Urinating
Dampness	Bowel movement
Weather change	Tension
Massage, vibrator	Bright lights
Pressure	Loud noises
Movement	Going to work
Standing	Sexual activity
Bending	Sneezing
Mild exercise	Coughing

30. Do you think your pain is due to something more serious or different from what your doctors have told you? What do you think is the cause?
31. Since your pain began, which of the following people have you seen for treatment and pain relief?

Acupuncturist	Faith healer
Allergist	General or family doctor
Anesthesiologist	Gynecologist/obstetrician
Cardiologist	Hypnotist
Chiropractor	Internal medicine
Clergyman	Neurologist
Dentist	Neurosurgeon
Dermatologist	Ophthalmologist (eyes)
Endocrinologist	Orthopedist (bones & joints)

Osteopath

Otorhinolaryngologist
(ear, nose and throat)

Physiatrist

Plastic surgeon

Psychiatrist

Psychologist

Radiologist

Surgeon (general)

Others (specify)

32. Have doctors ever suggested that your pain was imaginary or "all in your head"?
33. Have any doctors or nurses ever acted as if they thought you were faking?
34. How did your pain begin?
    (A) Accident at work
    (B) Accident at home
    (C) Other accident
    (D) At work but not accident
    (E) Following surgery
    (F) Following illness
    (G) Pain just began one day
    (H) Other reasons
35. Please describe briefly your answer to question number 34.
36. When did you first experience the pain for which you are now seeking help?
37. In what parts of the body did the pain begin? (Name all parts.)
38. Is the pain rarely present; present under certain conditions; frequently present; usually present; always present?
39. Describe your answer to question number 38.
40. Is the *intensity* of your pain always the same or is it sometimes worse?
41. Describe your answer to question number 40.
42. The following words describe degrees of pain severity: 1 = mild; 2 = uncomfortable; 3 = fairly severe; 4 = very severe, horrible; 5 = unbearable, excruciating.

Please choose the number of the word which best describes the following:
    (A) Your pain as it usually feels
    (B) Your pain *right now*
    (C) Your pain at its *worst*
    (D) Your pain when it hurts *least*
    (E) The *worst* toothache you ever had
    (F) The *worst* headache you ever had
    (G) The *worst* stomachache you ever had
    (H) The *worst* sunburn you ever had
    (I) The *worst* insect bite you ever had

43. Do you have trouble falling asleep? Never; sometimes; usually; always.
44. Do you take medicine to help you sleep? Never; sometimes; usually; always. What is the name of the medicine?
45. Does the pain frequently wake you at night? If yes, how many times on an average night? When it does wake you up, what do you usually do?
    (A) Empty bladder
    (B) Take medication
    (C) Sit up for a while
    (D) Other (describe)
46. What does your husband or wife do when you wake up at night? (Do not just say "nothing"—be specific.)
47. What activities bring on the pain or make the pain worse?
48. About how long after beginning this activity does it take for the pain to begin or become worse?
49. Does the pain stop if you quit doing these activities?
50. How many times a day do you have to stop what you are doing because of the pain?
51. How many times a day do you have to lie down because of the pain?
52. Do you have days when the pain is so bad that you stay in bed? If so, how often does this happen?
53. If I were there when you were in pain, what would I see and hear? How do others around you know when you are in pain? (Describe fully.)
54. When you are in pain, what does your husband or wife do?
55. Have you ever been operated on for your pain? Never; once; twice; three times; four times; five times; more than five times.
56. If you have had surgery, give date of last operation.
57. Did any operation bring relief from the pain?
58. What is the longest period of relief after an operation?
59. Have you ever had nerve blocks (injections) for the pain? If yes, how many?
60. Do you take medicine for relief of your pain? Is it medicine that your doctor ordered? Is it medicine that you decided to take yourself?
61. What medicines are you *now* taking for pain, what is the dosage, and how often do you take each one? When did you first begin taking this (these) medications?
62. What other medicines do you take for conditions other than pain? Indicate the dosage, frequency and date started.
63. How effective is the pain medication you take? Always takes pain

away; always lessens pain; usually takes pain away; usually lessens pain; frequently takes pain away; frequently lessens pain; no effect at all.

64. What is the *longest* time that your medicine relieves your pain?

65. If you are *not* working now and had no pain problem, would you plan to go back to work? Do you plan to go to the same job you had before your injury?

66. If you could have *any* job, what would you really like to do?

67. What do you want from medical treatment? (Be as specific as you can.)

68. What do you expect from treatment? (Be as specific as you can.)

69. Do you feel that the doctors who have treated you for your pain have been sympathetic and understanding? Very sympathetic; somewhat sympathetic; hardly sympathetic; not at all sympathetic.

70. How would you rate your overall satisfaction with the care and treatment you have received for your pain so far? Very satisfied; somewhat satisfied; barely satisfied; dissatisfied; very dissatisfied.

71. If your treatment here does not bring you relief, do you think you will try somewhere else?

Selected Pain Treatment Centers in the United States

The following list of pain-treatment centers is adapted from *Pain Clinic Directory: 1979*, compiled by the American Society of Anesthesiologists and the International Association for the Study of Pain. This is only a sampling of various pain-treatment centers; many highly qualified and excellent centers are not listed because of space limitations. This listing is presented for information purposes only, and no endorsement or recommendation should be assumed. If you have an interest in one of the centers, write the center in care of the Director of Chronic Pain Services.

ARIZONA

University of Arizona Pain
  Clinic
1501 N. Campbell Avenue
Tucson, AZ 85719

CALIFORNIA

University of California
  Pain Center
U.C.L.A. School of Medicine
Los Angeles, CA 90033

Pain Treatment Center
Scripps Clinic Medical
  Institution
10666 N. Terrey Pines Road
La Jolla, CA

Pain Center
City of Hope National
  Medical Center
1500 E. Duarte Road
Duarte, CA 91010

COLORADO

Pain Clinic
University of Colorado
 Medical Center
Denver, CO

FLORIDA

Chronic Pain Rehabilitation
 Center
Baptist Hospital of Miami
8900 S.W. 88th Street
Miami, FL 33176

University of Miami
School of Medicine
Department of Neurology
Miami, FL

GEORGIA

Pain Control Center
Emory University School of
 Medicine
1441 Clifton Road, N.E.
Atlanta, GA 30322

ILLINOIS

Low Back and Pain Clinic
Northwestern University
 Medical Center
Chicago, IL

INDIANA

Community Hospital
 Rehabilitation Center for
 Pain
1500 N. Ritter Avenue
Indianapolis, IN 46219

KENTUCKY

Pain Rehabilitation Clinic
University of Kentucky
 Medical Center
800 Rose Street
Lexington, KY 40506

LOUISIANA

Doctor's Hospital Pain Unit
Doctor's Hospital
Shreveport, LA

MARYLAND

Pain Treatment Center
Johns Hopkins Hospital
601 N. Broadway
Baltimore, MD 21205

Mensana Clinic
Greenspring Valley Road
Stevenson, MD 21153

MASSACHUSETTS

University of Massachusetts
 Medical Center
Pain Clinic
55 N. Lake Avenue
Worcester, MA 01605

MICHIGAN

Rehabilitation Center
22401 Foster Winter Drive
Southfield, MI 48075

MINNESOTA

Pain Clinic
Mayo Clinic
Rochester, MN 55901

MISSOURI

Howard County General
  Chronic Pain Clinic
Cedar Lane and Little
  Patuxent Parkway
Columbia, MO 65201

NEBRASKA

The Pain Clinic
Suite 123
7701 Pacific Street
Omaha, NE 68114

NEW JERSEY

Pain Clinic
New Jersey Medical School
Newark, NJ

NEW YORK

Pain Program
Hospital for Joint Diseases
  and Medical Center
1919 Madison Avenue
New York, NY 10035

Nerve Block Clinic and
  Neurology Clinic of
  Presbyterian Hospital
Vanderbilt Clinic
Columbia Presbyterian
  Hospital
622 W. 168th Street
New York, NY 10032

NORTH CAROLINA

Pain Clinic
Duke University Medical
  Center
Durham, NC

Pain Program
Charlotte Rehabilitation
  Hospital
1100 Blythe Boulevard
Charlotte, NC 28203

OHIO

Cincinnati General Hospital
Pain Program
234 Goodman Avenue
Cincinnati, OH 45267

Chronic Pain Service
University Hospital of
  Cleveland
2065 Adelbert Road
Cleveland, OH 44106

OREGON

Sacred Heart Hospital
1200 Alder Street
Eugene, OR 97401

PENNSYLVANIA

Pain Control Center of
  Temple University
Temple University Hospital
3401 N. Broad Street
Philadelphia, PA 19140

Pain Control Center
University of Pittsburgh
Presbyterian University
  Hospital
230 Lothrop Street
Pittsburgh, PA 15213

RHODE ISLAND

Institute for Behavioral
  Medicine
Summit Medical Center
Providence, RI

SOUTH CAROLINA

Chronic Pain Rehabilitation
  Program
Roger C. Peace Institute of
  Rehabilitative Medicine
Greenville Hospital System
701 Grove Road
Greenville, SC 29605

TENNESSEE

University of Tennessee
  Pain Clinic
66 N. Pauline Street
Memphis, TN 38105

TEXAS

Pain Evaluation and
  Treatment Center
University of Texas Health
  Science Center
Dallas, TX

Texas Institute for
  Rehabilitation and
  Research
1333 Moursund Avenue
Houston, TX 77030

UTAH

McKay Dee Hospital Center
3939 Harrison Boulevard
Ogden, UT 84403

VIRGINIA

University of Virginia
  Medical Center
Box 293
Charlottesville, VA 22902

WASHINGTON

Operant Program for
  Chronic Pain
Department of Rehabilitative
  Medicine
University Hospital
Seattle, WA

University of Washington
  Hospital
1959 N.E. Pacific Street
Seattle, WA 98105

WEST VIRGINIA

Marshall University School
  of Medicine
Appalachian Regional
  Hospital
Beckley, WV

WISCONSIN

Pain Management Unit
Rehabilitation Medicine
University of Wisconsin
  Hospital
Madison, WI 53706

Additional Selected Pain Treatment Centers

AUSTRALIA

St. Vincents Hospital
Darlinghurst, Sydney NSW

Sir Charles Gairdner Hospital
Pain Relief Clinic
Nedlands, Australia 6009

Oro-Facial Pain Clinic
Royal Melbourne Dental
  School
University of Melbourne
711 Elizabeth Street
Melbourne, Australia

CANADA

Department of Anaesthesia
  Pain Clinic
Victoria General Hospital
Halifax, Nova Scotia

Irene Eleanor Smythe Pain
  Clinic
Toronto General Hospital
Toronto, Canada

Centre Hospitalier
  del Université
Laval, Quebec

Pain Unit
Montreal Neurological
  Hospital
3801 University Street
Montreal, Quebec

UNITED KINGDOM

Centre for Pain Relief
Walton Hospital
Liverpool, England

National Hospital for Nervous
  Diseases
Queen Square
London, England WC1

Pain Clinic
Freedom Fields Hospital
Plymouth, Devon
England

Professional Organizations

Academy of Psychosomatic
  Medicine
Suite 202
70 W. Hubbard Street
Chicago, IL 60610

American Academy of
  Occupational Medicine
150 N. Wacker Drive
Chicago, IL 60606

American Association for
  the Advancement of
  Science
1515 Massachusetts Avenue,
  N.W.
Washington, DC 20005

American Association for
  the Study of Headaches
5252 N. Western Avenue
Chicago, IL 60625

American Dental
  Association
211 E. Chicago Avenue
Chicago, IL 60611

American Medical
  Association
535 Dearborn Street
Washington, DC 60610

American Nurses
  Association
2420 Pershing Road
Kansas City, MO 64108

American Occupational
  Therapy Association
6000 Executive Boulevard
Rockville, MD 20852

American Psychiatric
  Association
1700 18th Street, N.W.
Washington, DC 20009

American Psychological
  Association
1200 17th Street, N.W.
Washington, DC 20036

Arthritis Foundation
3400 Peachtree Street, N.E.
Atlanta, GA 30326

Biofeedback Society of
  America
University of Colorado
  Medical Center
Denver, CO 80202

International Association for
  the Study of Pain
Department of
  Anesthesiology, RN-10
University of Washington
Seattle, WA 98195

National Association of
  Social Workers
Suite 600
1425 H Street, N.W.
Washington, DC 20005

National Rehabilitation
  Association
Suite 1120
1522 K Street, N.W.
Washington, DC 20005

Index